MCQs for the FRCS Examinations
in Applied Basic Sciences

KU-825-872

DISPOSED OF FROM
CWM TAF LIBRARY
SERVICES 2024
NEWER INFORMATION
MAY BE AVAILABLE

This book is to be returned on or before
the last date stamped below.

21 DEC 1997

E03487

MCQs for the FRCS Examinations in Applied Basic Sciences

Questions in Anatomy, Physiology, Pathology and Surgery in General

John Pegington FRCS

S A Courtauld Professor of Anatomy
Department of Anatomy & Developmental Biology
University College London

Fred J Imms BSc MB BS PhD

Senior Lecturer in Physiology
Sherrington School of Physiology
United Medical and Dental Schools
(St Thomas's Campus) of Guy's and St Thomas's Hospital
London

David R Davies MB BS MRCS LRCP FRCPath

Reader in Histopathology & Honorary Consultant Histopathologist
United Medical and Dental Schools
(St Thomas's Campus) of Guy's and St Thomas's Hospital
London

Paul B Boulos MS FRCS Ed

Reader in Surgery & Consultant Surgeon
Department of Surgery
University College London

Edward Arnold
A division of Hodder & Stoughton
LONDON   BOSTON   MELBOURNE   AUCKLAND

EAST GLAMORGAN GENERAL HOSPITAL
CHURCH VILLAGE. near PONTYPRIDD

© 1993 Edward Arnold

First published in Great Britain 1993
Distributed in the Americas by Little, Brown and Company,
34 Beacon Street, Boston, MA 02180

British Library Cataloguing in Publication Data

Pegington, John
  MCQs for FRCS Examinations
  in Applied Basic Sciences
  I. Title
  616.007

ISBN 0-340-57317-1

All rights reserved. No part of this publication may be reproduced
or transmitted in any form or by any means, electronically or
mechanically, including photocopying, recording or any
information storage or retrieval system, without either prior
permission in writing from the publisher or a licence permitting
restricted copying. In the United Kingdom such licences are issued
by the Copyright Licensing Agency: 90 Tottenham Court Road,
London W1P 9HE.

Whilst the advice and information in this book is believed to be true
and accurate at the date of going to press, neither the author nor
the publisher can accept any legal responsibility or liability for any
errors or omissions that may be made. In particular (but without
limiting the generality of the preceding disclaimer) every effort has
been made to check drug dosages; however, it is still possible
that errors have been missed. Furthermore, dosage schedules are
constantly being revised and new side-effects recognized. For these
reasons the reader is strongly urged to consult the drug companies'
printed instructions before administering any of the drugs
recommended in this book.

Typeset in Univers by Anneset, Weston-super-Mare, Avon
Printed and bound in Great Britain for Edward Arnold, a division
of Hodder and Stoughton Limited, Mill Road, Dunton Green,
Sevenoaks, Kent TN13 2YA by St Edmundsbury Press, Bury St
Edmunds, Suffolk and Hartnoll Ltd, Bodmin, Cornwall.

Preface

Multiple choice questions (MCQs) are used in surgical examinations throughout the world, and in the United Kingdom the written paper for the basic science section of the FRCS examination is exclusively based on such questions. The candidate therefore must approach this examination with this format in mind.

There are two categories of MCQs the 'single best response type' and the 'determinate type'. In the first, a format widely used in North America, the candidate selects one correct answer out of five suggested solutions; several variations of this type are used in any one examination. In the United Kingdom FRCS examinations, however, the MCQs are of the 'determinate type'. Here the candidate is required to state in respect of each option whether or not it is a correct solution to the problem in the stem of the question. The 'Applied Basic Medical Science' paper consists of MCQs covering the fields of anatomy, physiology and pathology. In the Scottish examinations questions on basic 'surgery in general' are also used, and therefore questions of this sort have been included in this text. The result of the FRCS MCQ paper is used to determine whether or not a candidate proceeds to the oral part of the examination.

When testing yourself on questions in this book, give +1 for each correct answer, −1 for each incorrect response, and 0 for items you leave unanswered. In the 'determinate type' question, therefore, a 'don't know' solution will not result in loss of a mark, but an incorrect response will. The score for each question can therefore vary from −5 to +5. The pass mark in MCQ papers often puzzles candidates. It is in the end, as in all examinations, an arbitrary cut-off level, to a certain extent judged by the experience of the examiners. Other more objective indices, however, are used to temper this experience; the mean score of all the candidates sitting the examination, the standard deviation, and the distribution curve of the marks are all taken into consideration when setting the final pass mark. As a very rough guide, you may consider the 'pass:fail boundary' somewhere in the range of 40–45% if this is your first attempt at the questions, but you should do considerably better at the second attempt.

The authors acknowledge the expert help and guidance given by Dr W G Gransden, Senior Lecturer in Microbiology at UMDS, St Thomas's Campus, in the creation and composition of the questions on microbiology (136–145). We are indebted to Mr Chris Sym and Jane Pendjiky of the Photographic Unit in the Department of Anatomy and Developmental Biology at University College London for photographic work and to Churchill Livingstone, *Publishers*, for allowing us to use radiographs from 'Clinical Anatomy in Action'. Thanks go to the staff of Edward Arnold for their help and encouragement during the production of the book. It is extremely difficult to set a group of questions that do not have some ambiguities. The authors would be grateful to hear from readers who have comments, or criticisms, or those who wish to point out errors.

London,
1992

Contents

1 Anatomy

1 During its course through the thorax the right vagus nerve
   (a) lies against the trachea.
   (b) runs in front of the left lung root.
   (c) contains fibres from the nucleus ambiguus destined for abdominal viscera.
   (d) gives branches to the pulmonary plexus.
   (e) takes part in the formation of an oesophageal plexus.

2 The left coronary artery
   (a) arises from the wall of the anterior aortic sinus (Gray's Anatomy nomen-
       clature).
   (b) runs between the pulmonary trunk and the left auricular appendage.
   (c) may bifurcate or trifurcate.
   (d) gives a sinuatrial nodal branch from its main stem in over 65% of hearts.
   (e) supplies the atrioventricular nodal artery in over 80% of hearts.

3 The oesophageal opening in the diaphragm
   (a) conducts anastomotic vessels between gastric and oesophageal venous
       systems.
   (b) is strengthened by muscle fibres from the right crus.
   (c) conducts the phrenic nerves.
   (d) is usually found on CT at the vertebral level of L1.
   (e) conducts the vena azygos.

4 The left phrenic nerve
   (a) is the sole motor supply to the diaphragm.
   (b) contains sensory fibres.
   (c) runs in the groove between the left subclavian and common carotid arteries.
   (d) runs between fibrous pericardium and pleura.
   (e) may be accompanied by an accessory nerve.

1 (a) **True** The vagus lies directly against the trachea.
  (b) **False** The vagus runs behind the lung root.
  (c) **False** These fibres, although they join the vagus, are destined to supply skeletal muscle of the pharynx and larynx via pharyngeal and laryngeal branches.
  (d) **True** The vagus contributes to both anterior and posterior pulmonary plexuses.
  (e) **True** Most of the right vagus contributes to the posterior oesophageal plexus and hence becomes the posterior vagal trunk. It should be noted, however, that both trunks contain fibres from both vagus nerves.

2 (a) **False** It is the right coronary artery that arises from this sinus, the left arises from the left posterior sinus.

   Note: **Clinical** terminology of the cusps: right coronary (anterior), left coronary (left posterior) and non-coronary (right posterior). **Nomina Anatomica** gives a fetal position nomenclature of right, left and posterior.

  (b) **True** The stem of the left coronary artery is short and its course lies between these two structures.
  (c) **True** The left coronary artery usually bifurcates into circumflex and anterior interventricular arteries. The left diagonal branch of the anterior interventricular artery may, however, be large and arise directly from the main trunk of the left coronary artery giving a trifurcation.
  (d) **False** The sinuatrial nodal artery is usually a branch of the right coronary artery. In 35% (Hutchinson, 1978) it may arise from the left coronary, but then is a branch of the circumflex.
  (e) **False** The atrioventricular nodal artery arises from the right coronary in 80% of hearts (Hutchinson, 1978).

3 (a) **True** Oesophageal branches of the left gastric vein become an important portocaval anastomosis in cirrhosis of the liver.
  (b) **True** These fibres form one of the mechanisms for preventing oesophageal reflux.
  (c) **False** The opening conducts the vagal trunks.
  (d) **False** The opening is usually higher than this at T10.
  (e) **False** The vena azygos passes through the aortic opening.

4 (a) **True** It now seems certain that the diaphragm, including the crura, gains motor supply from the phrenic nerves.
  (b) **True** Sensory fibres supply the mediastinal pleura, fibrous and parietal serous pericardium and pleura and peritoneum related to the diaphragm. Irritation under the diaphragm produces referred pain in the shoulder (C3, C4 and C5).
  (c) **True** From this groove it runs onto the aortic arch.
  (d) **True** The nerve runs superficial to the fibrous pericardium.
  (e) **True** An accessory phrenic nerve, usually a branch of the nerve to subclavius, occasionally accompanies and joins the main nerve.

5 Use the following angiogram to answer the question: the catheter 'C' is in the right
   ventricle.

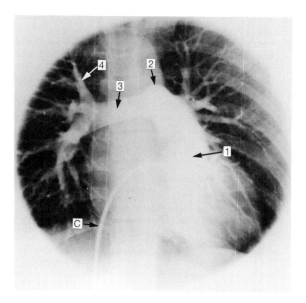

Fig. 1.1 Angiocardiogram. By kind permission of Churchill Livingstone, *Publishers.*
From *Clinical Anatomy in Action*, Volume 3: Pegington.

    (a) the vessel labelled '1' is enclosed within the pericardium.
    (b) vessel '1' is attached to the aortic arch at '2' by a ligament.
    (c) vessel '3' is related to the tracheal bifurcation.
    (d) vessel '3' is related to the cardiac plexus.
    (e) '4' is a segmental vessel.

6 The thymus
    (a) develops from the second pharyngeal pouch.
    (b) receives a blood supply directly from the subclavian artery.
    (c) has a supporting framework of strong collagenous tissue for lymphocytes
       within its lobules.
    (d) contains Hassal's corpuscles in the medulla of its lobules.
    (e) may be closely related to the inferior parathyroid in the adult.

5 (a) **True**   The pulmonary trunk is enclosed with the ascending aorta in a common tube of visceral pericardium.

   (b) **False**   Point '2' is the bifurcation of the pulmonary trunk, it is the **left** pulmonary artery that is attached to the arch by the ligamentum arteriousum.

   (c) **True**   The bifurcation of the pulmonary trunk '2' lies to the **left** of the tracheal bifurcation. The right pulmonary artery '3' therefore passes in front of the tracheal bifurcation and the right principal bronchus.

   (d) **True**   Much of the cardiac plexus is related to the tracheal bifurcation and, hence, the right pulmonary artery.

   (e) **False**   Vessel '4' is the right superior lobar artery. It usually divides into three segmental vessels.

6 (a) **False**   The gland develops from the third pouch: the tonsil grows from the second pouch.

   (b) **False**   The arterial supply comes from the internal thoracic and inferior thyroid arteries.

   (c) **False**   Unlike other lymphoid structures the thymic supporting tissue of the lymphocytes of the cortex and medulla consists mainly of epithelial cells.

   (d) **True**   These are formed by degenerating epitheliocytes that form concentric lamellae around a central mass.

   (e) **True**   Both glands develop from the third pharyngeal pouch, and an inferior parathyroid may descend into the thorax with the thymus.

7 Use the following CT of the chest to answer the following question.

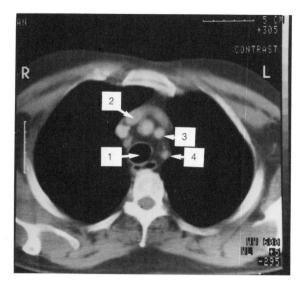

Fig. 1.2 CT of chest. By kind permission of Churchill Livingstone, *Publishers*. From *Clinical Anatomy in Action*, Volume 3: Pegington.

(a) the black area '1' is air in the oesophagus.
(b) the vessel '2' is a vein.
(c) vessel '3' is the brachiocephalic artery.
(d) some blood from vessel '4' is destined for the intracranial region.
(e) the level of the section is T5

8 Characteristics of cardiac myocytes are that
(a) they branch.
(b) they are multinucleate cells.
(c) they show striations similar to those of skeletal muscle fibres.
(d) they exhibit myogenic rhythm.
(e) they have intercalated discs between cells.

9 During a muscle splitting incision in the right iliac fossa for an appendicectomy the following structures will always be encountered:
(a) the membranous layer of superficial fascia.
(b) the rectus abdominis muscle.
(c) the aponeurosis of the external oblique.
(d) the ilioinguinal nerve.
(e) peritoneum.

7 (a) **False** The black area '1' is the trachea. Air can be seen in the oesophagus behind this structure.
   (b) **True** The brachiocephalic veins lie towards the front of the superior
mediastinum. Vessel '2' is the left brachiocephalic just above its
junction with the right vein which can be seen next to it.
   (c) **False** The brachiocephalic artery is to the right (subject's right) of '3': the
vessel in question is the left common carotid artery.
   (d) **True** Vessel '4' is the left subclavian artery, and one of its branches is
the vertebral artery.
   (e) **False** The section is taken above the aortic arch in the superior mediastinum, hence above the lower border of T4.

Note: The candidate should be able to identify the normal structures of the thorax on CT at three key levels: through the superior
mediastinum, at the aortic arch level and through the cavities of
the heart.

8 (a) **True** Each cell may branch into two or more branches at its ends.
   (b) **False** Cardiac cells are uninucleate.
   (c) **True** They have A, I, Z and H bands.
   (d) **True** An isolated cardiac myocyte contracts rhythmically although at a
rate slower than the normal heart.
   (e) **True** These consist of intermittent desmosomes and gap junctions.

9 (a) **True** The subcutaneous tissue in the lower abdomen consists of fatty
and membranous layers.
   (b) **False** A muscle splitting incision should not enter the rectus sheath.
   (c) **True** The split in the external oblique may be partly in muscle and
partly in aponeurosis, depending on the muscular development.
Muscular fibres usually end at a line from just below the umbilicus
to the anterior superior iliac spine.
   (d) **False** The nerve pierces the transversus and may be seen between this
muscle and the internal oblique. It is not actually encountered in
the standard muscle splitting incision, but may be damaged if the
incision is extended.
   (e) **True** Peritoneum must be incised to enter the peritoneal cavity.

10 The pyloric glands of the stomach
   (a) contain enteroendocrine cells.
   (b) are also known as Brunner's glands.
   (c) contain mucous cells.
   (d) contain chief (peptic) cells.
   (e) are the commonest site for oxyntic cells in the stomach.

11 Concerning mesenteries and other peritoneal folds
   (a) the left ureter is related to the sigmoid mesocolon.
   (b) the root of the mesentery (of the small intestine) crosses the second (descending) part of the duodenum.
   (c) the lower obliterated section of the lesser sac (omental bursa) lies between the two layers of the transverse mesocolon.
   (d) the paraduodenal fold contains an artery and a vein.
   (e) the ileocaecal fold (bloodless fold of Treves) lies behind the mesoappendix.

12 Structures that assist in the formation of the walls of the subphrenic peritoneal spaces (between diaphragm and transverse mesocolon) include
   (a) the suspensory ligament of the duodenum (ligament of Treitz).
   (b) the falciform ligament.
   (c) the superior leaf of the coronary ligament (of the liver).
   (d) peritoneum covering the right kidney.
   (e) the lesser omentum.

10 (a) **True**   The hormone gastrin is released by these cells in response to mechanical stimuli.

  (b) **False**   These glands are found in the submucous tissue of the duodenum.

  (c) **True**   These are found in the glands of all gastric areas; in the body and fundus special mucous (neck) cells are located at the necks of the glands.

  (d) **False**   These are found in main gastric glands of the body and fundus.

  (e) **False**   A few of these are usually found in the pyloric region although they are most plentiful in the glands of the body and fundus.

11 (a) **True**   The root of this mesentery is in the form of an inverted V and the left ureter descends into the pelvis behind its apex.

  (b) **False**   The root of the mesentery crosses the third part of the duodenum, the abdominal aorta, inferior vena cava and right ureter.

  (c) **False**   The embryological lesser sac extends between the layers of the greater omentum, but during development the layers become adherent.

  (d) **True**   The fold contains the inferior mesenteric vein and the ascending branch of the left colic artery.

  (e) **False**   The bloodless fold lies in front of the mesoappendix: it is not always bloodless.

12 (a) **False**   This mixed band of striated and smooth muscle assists in suspending the duodenojejunal flexure.

  (b) **True**   This lies between right and left subphrenic spaces above the liver.

  (c) **True**   This forms the posterior wall of the right subphrenic space above the liver.

  (d) **True**   This forms part of the wall of the right subhepatic subphrenic space (the hepatorenal pouch or pouch of Rutherford Morison).

  (e) **True**   The lesser sac (omental bursa) is one of the subphrenic spaces, and the lesser omentum is one of its walls.

13 Use this coeliac and superior mesenteric angiogram to answer this 'problem solving' question. 'C' is the loop of the catheter placed in the coeliac trunk. (L = liver; Vessel '3' = superior mesenteric artery)

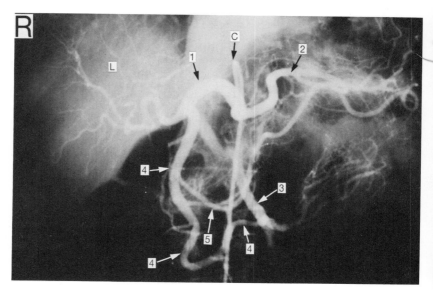

Fig. 1.3 Coeliac and superior mesenteric angiogram. By kind permission of Professor W D Jeans FRCR, MD, Professor of Radiology, Sultan Qaboos University, Sultantate of Oman.

(a) '1' is a vessel which normally bifurcates.
(b) '2' is a vessel which is closely related to the pancreas.
(c) '3' supplies branches to the duodenum.
(d) Vessel '4' (a branch of '3') supplies blood to the liver.
(e) '5' supplies blood to the stomach.

14 During surgical exposure of the right kidney through the lumbar approach below the twelfth rib, structures exposed may include
(a) pleura.
(b) lateral cutaneous nerve of thigh.
(c) the posterior edge of the external oblique.
(d) pararenal fascia.
(e) perirenal fat.

13 (a) **True**   '1' is the common hepatic artery. In this case it does not bifurcate and supplies the left lobe of the liver only, it thus becomes the left hepatic artery. This gives a clue to the interpretation of the rest of the angiogram.

(b) **True**   Vessel '2' is the splenic artery.

(c) **True**   The superior mesenteric artery gives the inferior pancreatico-duodenal artery, which supplies blood to the duodenum.

(d) **True**   In answer (a) it was noted that the hepatic artery did not give a right hepatic branch: '4' is an aberrant right hepatic artery arising from the superior mesenteric. Variations in gut vasculature are common and the candidate may be asked about common variations in the written and oral parts of the examination.

(e) **True**   '5' is the left gastro-epiploic branch, apparently arising directly from the aberrant right hepatic artery.

Note: Apart from identification of structures on a plane abdominal film and contrast films, the candidate should also be able to identify the abdominopelvic organs (liver, pancreas, spleen, suprarenals, uterus etc.) on CTs (For questions and examples see Pegington, J. *MCQs in Anatomy with answers and explanatory comments.* Sevenoaks: Edward Arnold, 1989, Figs 2.1, 2.3, 3.1 and 3.2.

14 (a) **True**   The lower edge of the pleura runs horizontally across the twelfth rib. It is more at risk if the twelfth rib is removed and the incision is made through its bed.

(b) **False**   This nerve is not a posterior relation of the kidney. The iliohypogastric and ilioinguinal nerves, although posterior relations should be at a lower level, although they may occasionally be seen. The subcostal neurovascular bundle will, however, be identified.

(c) **True**   The external oblique has a free posterior edge, unlike the internal oblique and transversus, which arise from lumbar fascia.

(d) **True**   This pad of fat is variable in size but is located behind the kidney external to the renal fascia.

(e) **True**   This layer of fat lies internal to the renal fascia, between it and the capsule of the kidney.

15 The appendix
  (a) is lined by villi.
  (b) is attached to the tip of a conical-shaped caecum in the new born infant.
  (c) has a complete coat of longitudinal muscle.
  (d) receives its blood supply from a vessel which runs behind the terminal ileum
      to reach the mesoappendix.
  (e) has a tip whose surface marking is known as McBurney's point.

16 During development of the midgut
  (a) a loop of gut enters the extra-embryonic coelom of the umbilical cord.
  (b) clockwise rotation occurs.
  (c) rotation occurs around the axis of the coeliac trunk.
  (d) a persistent vitelline (yolk) duct at the apex of the loop results in a Meckel's
      diverticulum.
  (e) the caecum is the last midgut structure to enter the abdomen.

17 The right colic flexure (hepatic flexure)
  (a) is related to the renal fascia of the right kidney.
  (b) forms part of the boundaries of the hepatorenal pouch.
  (c) is related to the horizontal (third) part of the duodenum.
  (d) is related to the right ureter.
  (e) is related to the neck of the gall bladder.

18 Structures lying behind the pancreas include
  (a) the lesser sac (omental bursa).
  (b) the right renal veins.
  (c) superior mesenteric vessels.
  (d) the portal vein.
  (e) the splenic vein.

15 (a) **False** Villi are characteristic of the small intestine: the appendix is lined with columnar epithelium.

(b) **True** In some cases this infantile state persists, but usually asymmetric growth of the caecum carries the base of the appendix to the posteromedial wall of the caecum.

(c) **True** The three taeniae of the large intestine become continuous at the appendicular base.

(d) **True** The lower division of the ileocolic artery gives the main blood supply to the appendix. Accessory vessels occur in 80% and an anastomotic vessel with the posterior caecal artery may be particularly large.

(e) **False** McBurney's point marks the position of the **base** of the appendix. Probably, however, the true surface marking is lower.

16 (a) **True** The loop enters the extra-embryonic coelom of the umbilical cord at the end of the fifth week. Re-entry occurs in the third month.

(b) **False** The rotation is counterclockwise.

(c) **False** Rotation occurs around the axis of the superior mesenteric artery.

(d) **True** This diverticulum projects from the antimesenteric border of the ileum about 1 m from the ileocaecal valve. It is found in 3% of subjects.

(e) **True** It subsequently reaches the right iliac fossa under a liver which is still relatively very large.

17 (a) **True** The posterior surface of the flexure is directly related to the renal fascia covering the kidney.

(b) **True** The other boundaries include the right lobe of the liver, the gall bladder, the right kidney and suprarenal and the descending part of the duodenum. See answer 12(d).

(c) **False** The flexure is related to the descending or second part of the duodenum.

(d) **False** At its origin the right ureter is overlapped by the descending (second) part of the duodenum.

(e) **False** The fundus, however, may be in contact with the flexure.

18 (a) **False** The lesser sac lies in front of the pancreas.

(b) **True** The head is related posteriorly to the inferior vena cava and the termination of both renal veins.

(c) **True** The vessels run behind the body of the pancreas and in front of the uncinate process.

(d) **True** This vessel lies behind the neck of the pancreas.

(e) **True** The vessel, at first contained in the lienorenal ligament with the artery and tail of the pancreas, is closely related to the posterior surface of body of the pancreas.

19 Posterior relations of the rectum include
  (a) peritoneum.
  (b) the promontory of the sacrum.
  (c) the sympathetic trunks.
  (d) the median sacral artery.
  (e) the fascia of Denonvilliers.

20 The prostatic part of the urethra
  (a) receives the ducts of the bulbourethral glands (Cowper).
  (b) is the narrowest part of the urethra.
  (c) is lined with stratified columnar epithelium.
  (d) contains branching mucous glands (of Littré).
  (e) receives the openings of the ducts of the seminal vesicles.

21 The vas (ductus) deferens
  (a) contains non-striated muscle in its walls.
  (b) arises from the head of the epididymis.
  (c) passes medial to the inferior epigastric artery.
  (d) crosses above the ureter as it approaches the bladder.
  (e) receives its blood supply from a branch of a vesical artery.

22 Concerning development of the urogenital system
  (a) the ureter develops from the paramesonephric (Müllerian) duct.
  (b) a horseshoe kidney is usually related to the inferior mesenteric artery.
  (c) in the adult the remnant of the urachus is known as the median umbilical ligament.
  (d) the convoluted tubules and loop of the nephron are formed from the ureteric bud.
  (e) an appendix of the testis is thought to be a remnant of the mesonephric duct.

19 (a) **False** Peritoneum is only related to the upper two-thirds of the rectum, covering the front and sides above and only the front lower down.

(b) **False** The rectum is related to the lower three sacral vertebrae and coccyx.

(c) **True** The trunks unite in front of the coccyx as the ganglion impar.

(d) **True** This is a branch of the aorta, a little above its bifurcation. Other posterior vascular relations are the lower lateral sacral vessels and branches of the superior rectal vessels.

(e) **False** This fascia is found between the rectum and the bladder, seminal vesicles and prostate. It is the fascia of Waldeyer that attaches the back of the rectum to the sacrum.

20 (a) **False** The glands lie below the prostate, close to the membranous urethra and their ducts open into the spongiose urethra almost 3 cm below.

(b) **False** The narrowest part lies at the external urethral orifice, followed by the membranous part.

(c) **False** The prostatic part of the urethra is lined with transitional epithelium: the rest of the male urethra is lined with stratified or pseudostratified columnar epithelium.

(d) **False** These are characteristic of the penile urethra.

(e) **False** Each seminal vesicle duct joins the ductus deferens to form an ejaculatory duct, and this duct opens into the prostatic urethra.

21 (a) **True** The thick muscle is arranged in external longitudinal and internal circular layers.

(b) **False** The vas arises at the tail of the epididymis and ascends along the back of the testis at the medial side of the epididymis.

(c) **False** At the deep inguinal ring the vas turns around the lateral side of this vessel.

(d) **True** In the female the uterine artery has a similar relationship to the ureter as it approaches the uterus.

(e) **True** This vessel anastomoses with branches of the testicular artery.

22 (a) **False** The ureter develops from the ureteric bud, an outgrowth from the mesonephric duct.

(b) **True** This type of kidney is prevented from abdominal ascent by the inferior mesenteric artery.

(c) **True** On each side of this fold the obliterated umbilical artery forms a medial umbilical ligament.

(d) **False** The ureteric bud forms the ureter, renal pelvis, calyces and collecting tubules: the glomerulus and tubules are formed from the metanephric mesoderm.

(e) **False** The appendix of the testis is thought to be a paramesonephric duct remnant.

23 In a transverse lower abdominal incision for access to the pelvis (Pfannenstiel's incision)
   (a) an incision is made through the anterior rectus sheath.
   (b) tendinous intersections of the rectus must be separated from the posterior rectus sheath.
   (c) the posterior layer of the rectus sheath must be divided.
   (d) the inferior epigastric vessels may be exposed if the rectus muscles are divided transversely.
   (e) the peritoneum must be incised in order to approach the prostate retropubically.

24 Ligaments or peritoneal folds having an attachment to the ovary include
   (a) the round ligament of the uterus.
   (b) the transverse cervical ligament (Mackenrodt).
   (c) the anterior leaf of the broad ligament.
   (d) the uterosacral ligament.
   (e) a remnant of the gubernaculum.

25 Concerning the sensory nerve supply and anaesthesia of the female external genitalia
   (a) the pudendal nerve may be approached by a needle directed into the greater sciatic foramen.
   (b) a pudendal nerve block results in anaesthesia of the anterior aspects of the labia majora.
   (c) some sensory nerve supply to the labium majus is obtained through the posterior femoral cutaneous nerve.
   (d) the ilioinguinal nerve supplies sensation to the clitoris.
   (e) a spinal anaesthetic at the level of the third sacral segment will result in anaesthesia of the entire labia majora.

26 The anorectal junction of the gut
   (a) is clearly demarcated by a line of anal valves.
   (b) obtains a blood supply from the superior rectal artery.
   (c) has a mucosa rich in goblet cells.
   (d) is sometimes known as Hilton's white line.
   (e) represents the junction between the endodermal and ectodermal parts of the lower gut.

23 (a) **True**   The anterior layers of the sheath may be opened in the line of the incision.

(b) **False**   Tendinous intersections are fused to the anterior layer of the rectus sheath, and are found near the umbilicus, close to the xiphoid and one midway between the two.

(c) **False**   There is no posterior layer below the arcuate line.

(d) **True**   The vessels run behind the rectus and may be exposed if the rectus is reflected laterally.

(e) **False**   The prostate may be approached retropubically through the retropubic pad of fat.

24 (a) **False**   This ligament attaches to the uterus.

(b) **False**   These ligaments stretch from the cervix to pelvic wall along fibrous tissue surrounding the uterine vessels.

(c) **False**   The mesovarium is attached to the posterior leaf of the broad ligament and thence to the ovary.

(d) **False**   The ligament stretches between the sacrum and cervix.

(e) **True**   The ovarian ligament is attached to the ovary and to the uterus close to the round ligament of the uterus. The two ligaments together represent the gubernaculum.

25 (a) **False**   The pudendal nerve may be approached by an injection on the medial side of the ischial tuberosity with the needle directed to the pudendal canal, or through the vaginal wall, the needle being directed to the ischial spine.

(b) **False**   The labial branches (scrotal branches in the male) only serve the posterior aspect of the labium (scrotum).

(c) **True**   Its perineal branches supply some sensation to the posterior labium and in the male to the back of the scrotum.

(d) **False**   The ilioinguinal nerve supplies the front of the labium (front of the scrotum in the male). The clitoris is supplied by the dorsal nerve arising from the pudendal nerve.

(e) **False**   The front of the labia (ilioinguinal and genitofemoral nerves) will require anaesthesia to the first lumbar level. A similar situation exists in the scrotum, the front being supplied from L1 and the back by S3.

26 (a) **False**   The junction is not clearly demarcated, and is defined as the level at which the gut passes through the pelvic diaphragm. The anal valves lie lower down **within** the anal canal proper.

(b) **True**   Below the line of the anal valves (pectinate line) the blood supply comes from the inferior rectal branch of the internal pudendal artery.

(c) **True**   The histological change from large bowel mucosa with goblet cells to non-keratinized stratified squamous epithelium occurs at a variable level above the pectinate line, but the upper canal has a mucosa similar to that of the rectum.

(d) **False**   This line lies below the pectinate line, and is simply an intersphincteric groove between the internal sphincter and the subcutaneous part of the external sphincter.

(e) **False**   It is generally accepted that the pectinate line represents this developmental junction.

27 In a lesion involving the motor nucleus of the **left** seventh cranial nerve
    (a) both left and right frontalis muscles function normally.
    (b) the left nasolabial fold is flattened.
    (c) the subject cannot close the left eye.
    (d) taste is lost over the anterior two-thirds of the tongue.
    (e) the subject suffers from left hyperacusis.

28 The abducent nerve (sixth cranial nerve)
    (a) is bathed in cerebrospinal fluid in part of its course.
    (b) travels close to the apex of the petrous temporal bone.
    (c) runs above the internal carotid artery during part of its course.
    (d) enters the orbit within the annular tendon.
    (e) supplies the superior oblique muscle of the orbit.

29 During surgical removal of a **left** submandibular gland
    (a) injury to the cervical branch of the facial nerve would result in loss of sensation over the angle of the mandible.
    (b) injury to the marginal mandibular branch of the facial nerve would result in drooping of the left angle of the mouth.
    (c) injury to the hypoglossal nerve will result in a deviation of the tongue to the right when the patient attempts to protrude it.
    (d) injury to the lingual nerve would result in loss of taste on the left anterior two-thirds of the tongue.
    (e) the great auricular nerve is at risk.

30 The middle meningeal artery
    (a) enters the skull through the foramen ovale.
    (b) supplies brain tissue.
    (c) runs a subdural course within the cranial cavity.
    (d) gives an anterior branch which runs deep to the pterion.
    (e) supplies blood to bones of the cranial vault.

27 (a) **False** In a lower motor neurone lesion the frontalis muscle on the side of the lesion is paralysed: in an upper motor neurone lesion, however, only the facial muscles below the eyes are affected because of the bilateral innervation of the upper face.

(b) **True** This results from paralysis of muscles of facial expression on the left.

(c) **True** This is a serious result and may require a tarsorrhaphy.

(d) **False** The fibres of the chorda tympani, carrying taste fibres from the anterior two-thirds of the tongue, have their cell bodies in the geniculate ganglion and their centripetal processes end in the nucleus solitarius.

(e) **True** Damage to the motor nerve to stapedius results in sounds appearing excessively loud; the function of the muscle is to dampen down sound waves.

28 (a) **True** Like other cranial nerves, the abducent nerve crosses the subarachnoid space; it runs through the pontine cistern and then enters the cavernous sinus below the petrosphenoidal ligament of Grüber, a ligament joining the dorsum sellae to the petrous apex.

(b) **True** Infections of the apical air cells can affect the nerve.

(c) **False** The nerve travels inferolateral to the artery through the cavernous sinus.

(d) **True** Other nerves within the circular tendon include the superior and inferior rami of the third nerve and the nasociliary nerve.

(e) **False** The nerve supplies the lateral rectus.

29 (a) **False** The candidate is advised to learn the relations of the major salivary glands and the dangers associated with surgery. The cervical branch is motor to the platysma.

(b) **True** This branch supplies the risorius and other muscles of the lower lip and chin.

(c) **False** Injury of a hypoglossal nerve results in deviation of the tongue to the side of the lesion.

(d) **True** The lingual nerve runs deep to the gland, and contains seventh nerve fibres for taste.

(e) **False** The course of this nerve takes it across the sternomastoid muscle and close to the parotid gland.

30 (a) **False** The artery enters the cranial cavity through the foramen spinosum.

(b) **False** The artery supplies no blood to nervous tissue.

(c) **False** The artery takes an extradural course.

(d) **True** The anterior branch lies deep to the pterion, the H-shaped sutural area made by the frontal, parietal, temporal and sphenoid bones.

(e) **True** The artery is a nutrient vessel to bone.

31 Use the following diagram to answer the question.

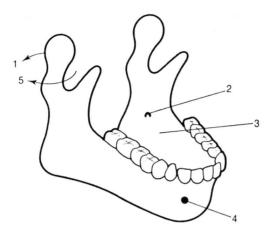

Fig. 1.4 Mandible viewed from the right.

With regard to nerves in close relation to the mandible
  (a) arrow '1' represents the course taken by the nerve to masseter.
  (b) a branch of the mandibular nerve enters the foramen in the mandible at '2'.
  (c) the hypoglossal nerve is directly related to the mandible at '3'.
  (d) the nerve that emerges at '4' supplies sensation over the chin.
  (e) arrow '5' represents the course taken by the buccal nerve.

32 When operating on a branchial fistula developed between the second pharyngeal pouch and cleft
  (a) the tract will be found passing in front of the common carotid artery.
  (b) its internal opening will be close to the tonsil.
  (c) the tract will be closely related to the glossopharyngeal nerve.
  (d) the hypoglossal nerve may be at risk during excision.
  (e) the external opening is likely to be somewhere in the posterior triangle of the neck.

31 (a) **False** It is the auriculotemporal nerve, which travels behind the neck of the mandible.

   (b) **True** The inferior alveolar nerve enters the bone through the mandibular foramen.

   (c) **False** It is the lingual nerve that is related to the bone near the roots of the third lower molar tooth.

   (d) **True** The mental nerve emerges through this foramen.

   (e) **False** This arrow represents the course taken by the nerve to masseter.

32 (a) **False** The tract runs in the fork between internal and external carotid arteries.

   (b) **True** The opening is usually in or near the intratonsillar cleft (supratonsillar fossa).

   (c) **True** The nerve passes between the internal and external carotids. The other two structures following this course between the vessels are the stylopharyngeus muscle and the pharyngeal branch of the vagus.

   (d) **True** The hypoglossal nerve embraces the carotid tree just above the bifurcation.

   (e) **False** The opening is usually situated along the anterior border of the sternocleidomastoid.

33 Use the mid-sagittal reconstruction CT scan of the upper cervical column to answer the question.

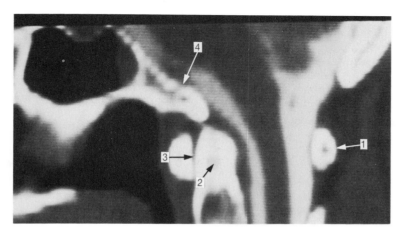

Fig. 1.5 CT of upper cervical column. By kind permission of Mr A Crockard FRCS and Mr A Jackovski FRCS, National Hospital for Nervous Diseases, Queen Square, London.

    (a) the vertebral artery runs below '1'.
    (b) the anterior longitudinal ligament is attached to '2'.
    (c) space '3' represents a primary catilaginous joint.
    (d) the sloping edge '4' is known as the clivus.
    (e) the named bony prominence '2' is completely ossified at birth.

34 A needle and catheter used for supraclavicular approach to the **left** subclavian vein
    (a) pierces the platysma.
    (b) may encounter a valve in the vein.
    (c) pierces scalenus anterior before entering the vein.
    (d) should enter the vein at its junction with the internal jugular vein.
    (e) will encounter the apex of the pleura before entering the vein.

33 (a) **False** Both the vertebral artery and the first cervical spinal nerve run **above** the posterior arch of the atlas. The CT is a mid-sagittal section and '1' is the posterior tubercle of the posterior arch.

(b) **False** Its upper end extends from the occipital bone to the anterior tubercle of the atlas and thence to the body of the axis: in whiplash lesion this latter attachment may be avulsed. It is not attached to the dens '2'.

(c) **False** The joint between the dens and the anterior arch of the atlas is synovial.

(d) **True** The clivus is formed from the fused basisphenoid and basiocciput. The primary cartilaginous joint between these bones fuses sometime during the late teens or early 20s.

(e) **False** Prominence '2' is the dens. It has an ossification centre at its tip which does not appear until the second year and which unites at about the age of 12 years. A translucent line is therefore visible on radiographs of the dens in young children.

34 (a) **True** Platysma lies in the subcutaneous tissue of the neck.

(b) **True** The subclavian vein usually has a pair of valves about 2 cm from its end. The internal jugular vein also contains valves, but the brachiocephalics are devoid of valves.

(c) **False** The vein runs in front of scalenus anterior.

(d) **False** The junction of the two veins is avoided; the thoracic duct enters the venous system in this position on the left side and may be damaged.

(e) **False** The apex of the pleura lies below and behind the vein.

35 Use the following lateral digital subtraction angiogram of the carotids to answer the following question. The catheter 'C' is in the external carotid artery.

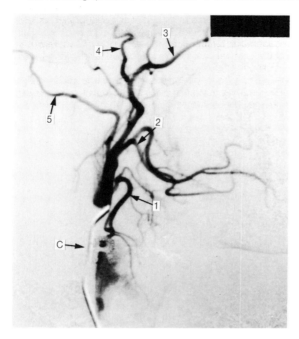

Fig. 1.6 Lateral digital subtraction angiogram. By kind permission of Professor W D Jeans FRCR, MD, Professor of Radiology, Sultan Qaboos University, Sultantate of Oman.

    (a) vessel '1' is related to the recurrent laryngeal nerve.
    (b) the loop in vessel '2' is related to a cranial nerve.
    (c) vessel '3' supplies a branch which enters the cranial cavity.
    (d) vessel '4' is related to a salivary gland.
    (e) vessel '5' is the posterior auricular artery.

36 Branches of the internal carotid artery include
    (a) the ophthalmic artery.
    (b) the anterior communicating artery.
    (c) hypophysial (pituitary) arteries.
    (d) the middle meningeal artery.
    (e) the middle cerebral artery.

35 (a) **False** '1' is the superior thyroid artery, and this is related to the external laryngeal nerve, a relationship important during thyroidectomy.

(b) **True** The loop of the lingual artery '2' is related to the hypoglossal nerve.

(c) **True** '3' is the maxillary artery and its middle meningeal branch enters the cranial cavity through the foramen spinosum.

(d) **True** '4' is the superficial temporal artery, one of the two terminal branches of the external carotid; the bifurcation takes place within the parotid gland.

(e) **False** Vessel '5' arising opposite the facial artery is the occipital artery. The posterior auricular vessel is small and can be seen on the angiogram above and parallel to '5'.

36 (a) **True** The vessel arises from the internal carotid just as it is about to leave the cavernous sinus and then enters the orbit through the optic canal.

(b) **False** This vessel joins the two anterior cerebral vessels: the posterior communicating artery is, however, a branch of the internal carotid.

(c) **True** There is usually one inferior and several superior arteries giving an important supply to the pituitary gland.

(d) **False** Although the artery may give a small meningeal branch, the middle meningeal is a branch of the maxillary artery.

(e) **True** This vessel and the anterior cerebral artery are the two terminal branches of the internal carotid.

37 Concerning the autonomic nervous system in the head and neck:
   (a) the stellate ganglion lies behind the vertebral artery.
   (b) damage to the autonomic fibres in the oculomotor nerve results in a constricted pupil.
   (c) the chorda tympani contains parasympathetic fibres.
   (d) the pharyngeal plexus receives a sympathetic input.
   (e) the geniculate ganglion contains parasympathetic synapses.

38 During thyroidectomy
   (a) the middle thyroid vein is found running in front of the common carotid artery.
   (b) the sternohyoid and sternothyroid muscles may be divided transversely in their upper ends to avoid injury to their nerve supply.
   (c) the recurrent laryngeal nerve may be located behind the cricothyroid joint.
   (d) damage to the external laryngeal nerve is most likely to occur when exposing the inferior thyroid artery.
   (e) a remnant of the thyroglossal duct may be found attached to the isthmus.

39 If the ulnar nerve is damaged behind the medial epicondyle
   (a) there will be loss of sweating from the skin of the hypothenar eminence.
   (b) there will be loss of sensation in the skin on the dorsum of the fifth metacarpal.
   (c) a 'trick' movement will be required to oppose the thumb to the index finger.
   (d) slight 'clawing' will be noted in the fourth and fifth digits.
   (e) adductor pollicis is paralysed.

37 (a) **True** The large ganglion lies behind the vertebral artery, in front of the neck of the first rib.

(b) **False** The parasympathetic fibres, derived from the Edinger–Westphal nucleus, synapse in the ciliary ganglion and supply the ciliary muscle and the constrictor pupillae. Damage to the third nerve therefore results in dilatation of the pupil; this is seen with the increased intracranial pressure of a severe head injury.

(c) **True** Preganglionic parasympathetic fibres from this nerve pass to the lingual nerve, synapse in the submandibular ganglion and postganglionic fibres innervate the submandibular and sublingual salivary glands.

(d) **True** The plexus is formed by the pharyngeal branch of the vagus (mainly motor fibres of the cranial accessory), the glossopharyngeal nerve (sensory) and sympathetic fibres (probably vasoconstrictor).

(e) **False** The geniculate ganglion is a sensory ganglion (taste) associated with the facial nerve.

38 (a) **True** The vessel crosses the common carotid and drains into the internal jugular vein.

(b) **True** The nerve supply from the ansa cervicalis is avoided if the muscles are transected high up.

(c) **True** The nerve passes in the groove between the trachea and oesophagus and then passes behind the ligament of Berry and the cricothyroid joint.

(d) **False** The external laryngeal nerve is related to the superior thyroid artery.

(e) **True** A thyroglossal tract remnant may extend from the foramen caecum of the tongue as far as the isthmus of the thyroid gland. Its relationship to the hyoid bone should also be noted, in that it descends at first in front of the bone and then takes a small loop upwards behind the bone before completing its descent.

39 (a) **True** Sympathetic fibres to sweat glands are carried in the cutaneous nerves; the ulnar nerve supplies skin over the hypothenar eminence.

(b) **True** The back of the hand over the fifth metacarpal is supplied by the dorsal cutaneous branch of the ulnar nerve.

(c) **False** Opposition is unaffected; the thenar eminence muscles are supplied by the median nerve.

(d) **True** 'Claw' hand results from an ulnar nerve lesion and affects mainly the fourth and fifth digits. The metacarpophalangeal joints are hyperextended and each of the interphalangeal joints flexed to a right angle. If the lesion is above the elbow, however, paralysis of the ulnar half of the flexor digitorum profundus (ring and little fingers) releases the flexion deformities of the interphalangeal joints and only slight clawing is evident.

(e) **True** This muscle is tested by means of Froment's test.

40 Concerning clinical examination in the upper limb:
   (a) in order to test the function of the axillary nerve following dislocation of the shoulder, sensation is tested over the tip of the shoulder.
   (b) the myotomes concerned in the elbow (biceps) reflex are C5 and C6.
   (c) in order to test the function of flexor digitorum superficialis in isolation from the profundus the subject is asked to flex the fingers around a soft ball.
   (d) one way of testing the function of biceps is to ask the subject to supinate the forearm with the elbow in the fully extended position.
   (e) abduction of the thumb at its metacarpophalangeal joint is a test of the motor component of median nerve function.

41 The scaphoid
   (a) receives nutrient vessels at its waist.
   (b) is closely related to the radial artery.
   (c) has a tubercle which may be palpated in the anatomical snuffbox.
   (d) articulates with the radius.
   (e) starts to ossify at birth.

42 The median nerve in the upper arm (axilla to the level of the epicondyles)
   (a) travels through the lower triangular space.
   (b) gives branches.
   (c) crosses in front of the brachial artery and its venae comitantes.
   (d) carries parasympathetic fibres.
   (e) communicates with the ulnar nerve.

40 (a) **False** Supraclavicular nerves supply the skin of the shoulder tip: the territory for the axillary nerve is lower, over the lower deltoid or 'badge' area – so called because it is here that scouts wear their badges.

(b) **True** The myotomes involved in reflexes are particularly important for the candidate to learn.

(c) **False** To perform this test the hand is placed with its dorsum flat on a table and the other three fingers of the hand are held with their dorsal surfaces against the table. Only the finger under examination is left free to flex, and on doing this it flexes at the proximal joint (flexor dig.sup. function).

(d) **False** Biceps is a powerful supinator with the elbow flexed to a right angle; it does not perform this function with the elbow in the straight position.

(e) **True** The best way to test the function of abductor pollicis brevis is to place the dorsum of the hand against a table and ask the subject to raise the tip of the thumb towards a pen held above – 'pen touching test'.

41 (a) **True** Nutrient vessels enter the non-articular sections of the bone – the waist and the tubercle, especially on the dorsal surface. Fracture through the waist may result in avascular necrosis of the proximal pole of the bone.

(b) **True** The radial artery runs through the base of the anatomical snuffbox and gives nutrient branches to the bone.

(c) **False** It is the waist which is palpated in the anatomical snuffbox: the tubercle is palpated in front of the snuffbox.

(d) **True** The bone articulates with a triangular articular surface on the radius.

(e) **False** The carpus is cartilaginous at birth: the first of the carpal bones to ossify is the capitate closely followed by the hamate during the first few months. The order of the remaining bone ossification varies, but the scaphoid usually starts at 4–5 years.

42 (a) **False** It is the radial nerve which goes through this space.

(b) **True** Although denied in some texts, vascular branches go to the brachial artery and usually there is also a branch to pronator teres given off above the elbow.

(c) **True** This is the usual course, although it may rarely pass behind the vessels.

Note: What do you know about venae comitantes? Read the introductory chapters in Last's Anatomy Regional & Applied and Grant's Method of Anatomy; these contain a wealth of basic anatomical information.

(d) **False** It does, however, carry sympathetic fibres which innervate blood vessels, sweat glands and arrector pili muscles.

(e) **True** This item tests the very good students: C7 fibres from the median nerve join the ulnar nerve. Communicating branches are frequently found between nerves, e.g. between cranial nerves, cranial nerves and the sympathetic trunk at the skull base and between branches of the facial nerve and sensory nerves on the face.

43 Concerning normal and abnormal joint alignment in the limbs:
  (a) the angle of inclination in the femur is increased in coxa vara.
  (b) there is normally a varus angle of 8° at the knee joint.
  (c) abductor hallucis opposes the deformity of hallux valgus.
  (d) shortening of the tendo calcaneus results in talipes calcaneovalgus.
  (e) a physiological varus angle at the elbow is known as the 'carrying' angle.

44 The first lumbrical muscle
  (a) arises from the second metacarpal.
  (b) is bipennate.
  (c) passes to the radial side of the index finger.
  (d) contains a sesamoid bone.
  (e) inserts into the proximal phalanx of the index finger.

43 (a) **False** The angle of inclination is the angle between the shaft and neck of the femur. The candidate should know the definitions of the terms 'varus' and 'valgus'. The former defines a joint deformity which results in the distal end of the limb approaching the body, and the latter a deformity which carries it away from the body. 'Coxa' is the name for the hip. In Fig 1.7, the first diagram shows the normal angle, the second coxa vara and the third coxa valga.

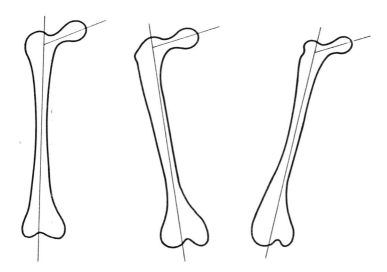

Fig. 1.7 The angle of inclination.

(b) **False** There is a valgus angle of this degree at the knee.
(c) **True** The abductor is the only muscle capable of opposing the development of the deformity.
(d) **False** Shortening of the tendo calcaneus results in a plantarflexion deformity at the ankle known as 'equinus': a dorsiflexion deformity is 'calcaneus'. Club foot is talipes (ankle) equino-varus.
(e) **False** The carrying angle at the elbow is a valgus angle.

44 (a) **False** The lumbricals arise from the tendons of flexor digitorum profundus.
(b) **False** Although variations occur, it is usually the third and fourth lumbricals that are bipennate.
(c) **True** All four lumbricals run on the radial side of their respective finger.
(d) **False** Sesamoid bones are associated with the small muscles of the thumb, not the lumbricals.
(e) **False** It inserts into the dorsal expansion of the index.

45 During an anterolateral approach to the hip joint
    (a) access is gained in the interval between gluteus medius and gluteus maximus.
    (b) a branch of the lateral femoral circumflex artery will be exposed.
    (c) the inferior gluteal nerve is at risk in the operating field.
    (d) the reflected head of rectus femoris is exposed.
    (e) the tendon of obturator externus will be exposed running on the front of the femoral neck.

46 Concerning the upper end of the developing femur:
    (a) the ossification centre for the head lies at the 'growing end' of the femur.
    (b) the ossification centre for the head is visible on a radiograph of the hip of a newborn infant.
    (c) the epiphysis for the lesser trochanter is an atavistic type.
    (d) the metaphysis lies adjacent to the growth disc (epiphysial plate).
    (e) the epiphysial bone receives blood from the obturator artery.

47 Ligaments forming part of the boundaries of the femoral ring include
    (a) the reflected part of the inguinal ligament.
    (b) the lacunar ligament.
    (c) the interfoveolar ligament.
    (d) the inguinal ligament.
    (e) the pectineal ligament.

45 (a) **False** The applied anatomy involved in the standard approaches to the hip is a good test of the candidate's grasp of this region. The **anterior approach** is through the interval between tensor and sartorius, and the **anterolateral** between tensor and gluteus medius. The iliotibial tract is incised over the greater trochanter in the **lateral** approach, and the **posterior** approach involves splitting gluteus maximus in the line of its fibres.

(b) **True** The ascending branch of this vessel runs deep to tensor and gluteus medius, and will therefore be found as the interval between these muscles is exposed.

(c) **False** This supplies gluteus maximus; the nerve to the tensor is, however, at risk because it is found in the gap between tensor and gluteus medius.

(d) **True** This is attached to the upper acetabular rim.

(e) **False** The tendon of obturator externus runs along the back of the femoral neck.

46 (a) **False** The so-called growing end of a long bone is the last of the two end epiphyses to unite, and, apart from the fibula, it is also the first to appear. In the femur the lower end is the first to appear (at birth) and unites later than the epiphysis at the upper end.

(b) **False** The epiphysis for the head of the femur is first seen towards the end of the first year of life.

(c) **False** There are three types of epiphyses. An atavistic epiphysis represents a skeletal element separate at an earlier stage of evolution: the small centre at the apex of the coracoid process is an example. The end epiphyses of long bones are known as pressure epiphyses and those resulting from muscle pull, such as the trochanteric epiphyses, are traction epiphyses.

(d) **True** The metaphysis is that part of the diaphysis next to the growth disc: it is the section of bone commonly affected in osteomyelitis.

(e) **True** The developing head receives blood from a branch of this vessel, which reaches it via the ligamentum teres.

47 (a) **False** The reflected part of the inguinal ligament is an expansion from the medial attachment of the inguinal ligament. It passes upwards and medially to reach the rectus sheath and linea alba.

(b) **True** This is the medial boundary of the ring and may be incised to release an obstruction at the neck of a femoral hernia. An abnormal obturator artery, an enlarged pubic branch of the inferior epigastric artery, which is found in 30% of individuals, usually descends lateral to the femoral ring, but occasionally runs on the deep surface of the ligament medial to the ring.

(c) **False** This inconstant structure connects the lower margin of the transversus abdominis to the superior pubic ramus.

(d) **True** This is the anterior boundary of the ring.

(e) **True** This forms the posterior boundary and is strong enough to hold sutures used in a hernia repair.

48 Use the following arteriogram to answer the question. 'P' is the posterior tibial artery.

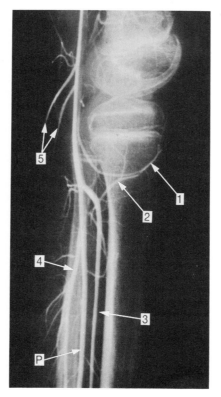

Fig 1.8 Popliteal angiogram. By kind permission of Professor W D Jeans FRCR, MD, Professor of Radiology, Sultan Qaboos University, Sultantate of Oman.

(a) vessel '1' is related to a ligament.
(b) vessel '2' is the anterior tibial recurrent artery.
(c) vessel '3' is related to the deep peroneal nerve.
(d) vessel '4' is the peroneal artery.
(e) vessels '5' supply the cruciate ligaments.

48 (a) **True**   This vessel is the inferior medial genicular artery, and runs deep to the tibial collateral ligament.

  (b) **True**   This vessel forms part of the genicular anastomosis.

  (c) **True**   Once the anterior tibial artery '3' passes through the interosseous membrane it is joined on its lateral side by the deep peroneal nerve.

  (d) **True**   This branch of the posterior tibial artery supplies muscles, a nutrient artery to the fibula and branches in the ankle region.

  (e) **False**   These vessels do not enter the knee joint but are muscular (sural) branches, often two in number and large, which supply gastrocnemius and soleus.

49 Use the following diagram to answer the question.

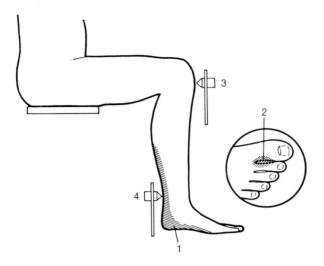

Fig. 1.9 Lateral view of leg and foot.

(a) area '1' outlines the dermatome of S1.
(b) area '2' is supplied by the superficial peroneal nerve.
(c) the reflex at '3' tests L2, L3 myotomes.
(d) the reflex at '4' tests S1, S2 myotomes.
(e) dorsiflexion of the big toe tests S1.

50 Structures directly related to or attached to the lateral malleolus include
(a) the calcaneofibular ligament.
(b) the great saphenous vein.
(c) the deep peroneal nerve.
(d) the flexor retinaculum.
(e) the common synovial sheath of the peroneal tendons.

49 (a) **True**   Of the lower limb dermatomes S1 is particularly important; disc lesions often give symptoms in its distribution.

(b) **False**   This small area at the fork of the big and second toes is supplied by the deep peroneal nerve.

(c) **False**   Myotomes involved in reflexes are particularly important for the candidate to learn: the knee jerk tests L3, L4.

(d) **True**   The ankle jerk tests S1, S2.

(e) **True**   It is useful to remember that extensor hallucis longus is supplied through L5.

50 (a) **True**   The lateral ligament of the ankle is made up of anterior and posterior talofibular ligaments and the calcaneofibular ligament. It is the first of these which is commonly injured during an ankle sprain. In more severe injuries, rupture of the calcaneofibular ligament leads to ankle instability, and attempts at inverting the ankle lead to tilting of the talus in its mortice.

(b) **False**   The vein runs on the front of the medial malleolus.

(c) **False**   The closest nerve is the sural nerve which runs between the malleolus and the calcaneus.

(d) **False**   It is the superior peroneal retinaculum which is attached to this malleolus.

(e) **True**   The tendons of peroneus longus and brevis run in a common synovial sheath behind the malleolus. The brevis is the closer of the two to the malleolus.

2 Physiology

51 Production of normal erythrocytes (rbcs) is
   (a) reduced immediately following gastrectomy.
   (b) depressed in renal failure.
   (c) increased by injecting folate into a normal person.
   (d) depressed in a normal pregnancy.
   (e) increased by removal of a normal spleen.

52 Macrocytic anaemia may
   (a) occur in pregnancy.
   (b) be caused by a rapidly growing neoplasm.
   (c) occur in renal failure.
   (d) appear 2 years after gastrectomy.
   (e) result from iron deficiency.

53 The following is a safe and effective anticoagulant **both** for *in vitro* samples for laboratory investigations and in the body
   (a) citrate.
   (b) warfarin.
   (c) heparin.
   (d) oxalate.
   (e) vitamin K.

54 In the coronary circulation to the left ventricle
   (a) flow is greater in systole than in diastole.
   (b) the venous effluent is at least 70% saturated with oxygen when the body is at rest.
   (c) the flow increases in proportion to the product of cardiac output and mean arterial blood pressure.
   (d) noradrenaline causes vasoconstriction.
   (e) the flow is greater than to the right ventricle.

51 (a) **False** The body has several years stores of Vitamin B_{12}.
   (b) **True** The normal kidney produces erythropoietin which stimulates rbc production. In renal failure the haemoglobin concentration is usually below 50% of normal.
   (c) **False** Supranormal levels of folate do not enhance red cell production if it is already normal.
   (d) **False** The 'anaemia' of pregnancy is dilutional.
   (e) **False** Enlarged spleens may depress rbc production, but not normal spleens.

52 (a) **True** Pregnant women often become folate deficient because of the demands of the rapidly growing foetus.
   (b) **True** Tumours have a high requirement for folate.
   (c) **False** Erythropoietin levels are depressed in renal failure causing a normocytic anaemia.
   (d) **True** Vitamin B_{12} absorption will be reduced following removal of the tissue producing intrinsic factor, but the body has large reserves of the vitamin and the onset of anaemia is delayed.
   (e) **False** Iron deficiency causes microcytic anaemia.

53 (a) **False** Citrate chelates calcium ions and is effective *in vitro* but when citrated blood is administered to a patient the citrate is rapidly metabolized.
   (b) **False** Warfarin is a vitamin K antagonist and depresses the formation of clotting factors (especially prothrombin) in the liver. It cannot be effective if added to a blood sample *in vitro*.
   (c) **True** Heparin is a natural compound, which blocks the clotting cascade at several sites.
   (d) **False** Oxalate precipitates calcium as insoluble calcium oxalate and therefore cannot be administered to the body.
   (e) **False** Vitamin K is the precursor of several clotting factors and is not an anticoagulant.

54 (a) **False** During systole vessels are compressed by the myocardium thus reducing flow. It rises during diastole.
   (b) **False** By contrast with most organs the venous blood is only about 25% saturated with oxygen in the resting person.
   (c) **True** This is an approximate index of cardiac work. Since little extra oxygen can be removed from the blood [see (b)], then flow increases with work rate.
   (d) **False** This would be a disastrous situation.
   (e) **True** The work done by the right ventricle is much less.

55 When arterial blood passes through systemic capillaries
  (a) the haemoglobin concentration increases.
  (b) the concentration of chloride ions in red cells increases.
  (c) the pH of the plasma rises.
  (d) the fall of PO_2 increases the buffering capacity of haemoglobin.
  (e) on average 70–75% of the oxygen carried by haemoglobin diffuses into tissues.

56 Systemic veins
  (a) have a lower compliance than arteries.
  (b) are innervated by sympathetic constrictor fibres.
  (c) contain more than 60% of the blood volume.
  (d) within the chest may contain blood at a pressure less than atmospheric.
  (e) draining a limb have a greater total cross-sectional area than the arteries supplying it.

57 Blood flow in the hand will increase
  (a) when the subject stands.
  (b) when the feet are placed in cold water.
  (c) when the ulnar, radial and median nerves are blocked with local anaesthetic.
  (d) during a haemorrhage.
  (e) whilst the subject exercises in the heat.

58 In the pulmonary circulation
  (a) there is a higher resistance to flow than in the systemic circulation.
  (b) when the person is standing, flow is greater at the base of the lung than at the hilum.
  (c) adaptations to alterations in cardiac output occur through changes in vascular tone induced by the autonomic nervous system.
  (d) the arterioles constrict in response to a lowered oxygen tension in the surrounding alveoli.
  (e) there is little formation of interstitial fluid.

55 (a) **True** The volume of fluid filtered to the interstitial space exceeds that reabsorbed. The balance returns to the circulation through the lymphatic system.

(b) **True** Bicarbonate ions formed in the cell are exchanged for chloride ions from the plasma.

(c) **False** Increased PCO_2 lowers pH. This fall is not completely buffered by bicarbonate ions leaving the red cell.

(d) **True** Haemoglobin is a weaker acid than oxyhaemoglobin and therefore a better buffer.

(e) **False** This would occur in the coronary vessels at rest and in muscle during severe exercise. In most tissues about 20–25% of the oxygen is given up by haemoglobin.

56 (a) **False** Veins are thin walled and easily distended.

(b) **True** These may play important roles in control of venous capacity and of venous return.

(c) **True** Only a small percentage of the blood volume is in the heart and arterial vessels.

(d) **True** Veins run next to the pleural space which has a sub-atmospheric pressure.

(e) **True** The cross-sectional area of the veins is greater than that of the corresponding arteries, and blood flows more slowly in veins.

57 (a) **False** Cardiac output falls and there is reflex vasoconstriction to maintain blood pressure.

(b) **False** This leads to body core cooling and there is reflex constriction of the skin blood vessels.

(c) **True** These nerves contain many of the sympathetic fibres to the hand. The blocks will largely abolish sympathetic vasoconstrictor tone.

(d) **False** The fall in blood pressure results in reflex vasoconstriction.

(e) **True** Exercise in the heat will raise heat production and induce vasodilatation in the skin.

58 (a) **False** Remember: $$Resistance = \frac{Pressure}{Flow}$$
Flow is the same in the two circulations, but pressure is much lower in the pulmonary circulation.

(b) **True** In the standing subject, gravity induces a graded flow which is low at the apex and high at the base of the lung.

(c) **False** The pulmonary circulation adapts passively to changes of cardiac output.

(d) **True** Pulmonary arterioles constrict in response to lowered oxygen tension and thus reduce perfusion of underventilated areas of the lung. Systemic vessels dilate in response to local hypoxia.

(e) **True** Pulmonary capillary pressure is lower than colloid osmotic pressure.

59 Heart rate in the resting, supine subject may be increased by
   (a) passively raising the legs.
   (b) an injection of atropine.
   (c) exposure of the lower body to subatmospheric pressure.
   (d) sustaining a strong handgrip contraction.
   (e) regular and vigorous exercise.

60 Breathing a gas mixture containing 30% O_2, 5% CO_2 and 65% N for a few minutes will
   (a) increase ventilation.
   (b) increase arterial oxygen content by almost 50%.
   (c) shift the oxygen dissociation curve to the left.
   (d) induce a metabolic acidosis.
   (e) reduce the pH of the cerebrospinal fluid.

59 (a) **True** This temporarily increases venous return and thus raises atrial pressure. Stimulation of atrial stretch receptors cause reflex increase of heart rate (the Bainbridge reflex).

(b) **True** This will abolish vagal tone and increase the rate of firing of the pacemaker.

(c) **True** This is the 'suck box' test which causes pooling of blood in the lower body and simulates a postural change or haemorrhage.

(d) **True** Isometric exercise, as exemplified by a handgrip contraction, accelerates the heart through its sympathetic supply.

(e) **False** A period of training increases the stroke volume of the heart and therefore reduces the resting heart rate.

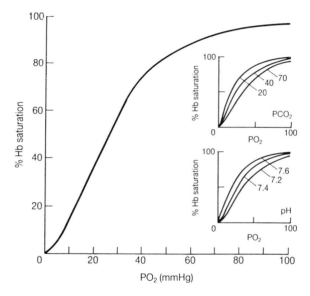

Fig. 2.1 The oxygen dissociation curve and (insets) shifts with changes in PCO_2 and pH.

60 (a) **True** The raised P_ICO_2 will raise P_ACO_2 and stimulate both peripheral and central chemoreceptors. Raising P_IO_2 will not appreciably suppress this response.

(b) **False** Haemoglobin during air breathing is at least 95% saturated. The amount of dissolved oxygen will increase by less than 0.2 ml dl^{-1} (Fig. 2.1).

(c) **False** Raising PCO_2 of blood shifts the oxygen dissociation curve to the right (Fig. 2.1).

(d) **False** Raising PCO_2 in blood causes a respiratory acidosis.

(e) **True** CO_2 diffuses rapidly into cerebrospinal fluid and forms carbonic acid.

61 In left ventricular failure there may be
  (a) peripheral cyanosis.
  (b) dilatation of the left ventricle.
  (c) breathlessness on exertion.
  (d) pulmonary oedema.
  (e) dyspnoea on lying flat.

62 Functional residual capacity
  (a) includes the residual volume.
  (b) is reduced in exercise.
  (c) PCO_2 rises during inspiration.
  (d) can be measured by rebreathing from a spirometer containing a known volume and concentration of helium.
  (e) will be increased if respiratory gas is applied at greater than atmospheric pressure.

63 A tension pneumothorax
  (a) causes further collapse of the lung with each inspiratory effort.
  (b) will displace the mediastinum to the non-affected side.
  (c) will lower the PO_2 of arterial blood.
  (d) is always due to air entering the pleural space from the lung.
  (e) may contain gas above atmospheric pressure.

64 The potassium ion concentration
  (a) in urine is less than 10% of the sodium concentration.
  (b) is low in adipose tissue.
  (c) rises in the plasma during exercise.
  (d) is low in the cerebrospinal fluid following head injury.
  (e) is greater in extracellular fluid than in intracellular fluid.

61 (a) **True**   When cardiac output is very low stagnant cyanosis may occur in peripheral capillaries.

(b) **True**   As the myocardium progressively fails and filling pressure rises, the ventricle becomes dilated.

(c) **True**   The patient is unable to raise cardiac output during exercise.

(d) **True**   A sequel to the raised filling pressure of the left ventricle.

(e) **True**   This is the symptom called orthopnoea. Lying flat increases venous return and hence the output of the right ventricle. The failing left ventricle cannot meet this demand until its filling pressure rises. This results in a high intravascular volume in the lungs and pulmonary oedema.

62 (a) **True**   Functional residual capacity comprises the expiratory reserve and residual volumes of the chest.

(b) **True**   Larger tidal volume encroaches on the expiratory reserve volume.

(c) **False**   During inspiration the functional residual capacity is diluted with atmospheric air.

(d) **True**   If V is the volume of gas in the spirometer and x_1 and x_2 the concentrations of helium in the spirometer before and after rebreathing, then $Vx_1 = (V + FRC)x_2$.

(e) **True**   Positive pressure breathing will distend the chest passively and expiration will be an active process against the inflation pressure.

63 (a) **True**   The tissue flap allows air to enter the pleural space during inspiration but prevents it from leaving during expiration.

(b) **True**   Increased volume in one pleural space will displace the mediastinum.

(c) **True**   Initially oxygenation will be impaired in the partially collapsed lung, but the reduced PO_2 will have only a small effect on oxygen content of mixed pulmonary venous blood. Later when the volume of air in the pneumothorax rises sufficiently to restrict air entry into both lungs then hypoxia becomes severe.

(d) **False**   The wound may be either in the lung or the chest wall.

(e) **True**   Particularly during expiration as air is compressed by the expiratory effort.

64 (a) **False**   The concentration of sodium and potassium in the urine do not reflect the relative concentrations in plasma. Since dietary intake of the ions is similar, the rates of excretion will be similar.

(b) **True**   Adipocytes contain little intracellular water and therefore little potassium.

(c) **True**   Potassium leaves cells during exercise and the arterial plasma concentration may rise 1 mmol in moderate exercise. The raised $[K^+]$ may play a role in stimulating ventilation in exercise.

(d) **False**   It is higher than normal because the homeostatic control of CSF and extracellular fluid composition is lost when the brain is injured.

(e) **False** $[K^+]$ is higher in intracellular fluid.

65 Oedema
    (a) of the ankles during standing will be greater in hot weather.
    (b) is part of the inflammatory response.
    (c) represents a marked increase of intracellular fluid volume.
    (d) is not a feature of liver failure.
    (e) of a region is likely to follow restoration of the circulation after prolonged ischaemia of the part.

66 Dialysis of a patient in renal failure can be used to temporarily correct
    (a) the plasma urea concentration.
    (b) the patient's acid–base status.
    (c) the nutritional state of the patient.
    (d) anaemia.
    (e) extracellular volume.

67 A metabolic acidosis occurs
    (a) in prolonged vomiting.
    (b) during ascent to altitude.
    (c) in renal failure.
    (d) in uncontrolled diabetes mellitus.
    (e) in hypokalaemia.

68 Rapid intravenous infusion of **one** litre of saline (154 mM) will
    (a) in a normal person lower the haemoglobin concentration.
    (b) in a person who has lost **one** litre of blood, maintain blood pressure for several hours.
    (c) be eliminated more slowly in a patient who underwent major surgery in the previous 24 hours.
    (d) in a normal person will be eliminated as quickly as **one** litre of water taken by mouth.
    (e) cause vasodilation in the vascular bed of muscle.

65 (a) **True** Under cool conditions oedema of the feet during standing is largely prevented by a major reduction of bloodflow. Bloodflow will increase during hot weather and increase the oedema.

(b) **True** The permeability of capillaries to protein is increased in inflammation.

(c) **False** Usually there is isotonic expansion of the extracellular fluid volume, and there is little osmotic movement of water across the cell membrane.

(d) **False** Liver failure lowers the plasma albumen concentration.

(e) **True** Ischaemia will lead to accumulation of metabolites in the interstitial fluid and will also increase capillary permeability.

66 (a) **True** Small molecules pass across the semi-permeable membrane and down a concentration gradient.

(b) **True** Fixed acid anions can be dialysed out and replaced by bicarbonate ions.

(c) **False** In theory, small amounts of glucose could enter the patient, but significant amounts of nutrients could not be given by this route.

(d) **False** Haemoglobin concentration may be slightly raised by reducing plasma volume, but the patient requires erythropoietin to stimulate red blood cell production by the bone marrow.

(e) **True** Using a slightly hypertonic dialysis fluid will withdraw water from the body.

67 (a) **False** Production of acid in the stomach is associated with passage of bicarbonate into plasma and a transient alkalosis, which is corrected when alkaline juices are secreted lower in the gastrointestinal tract. If acid is vomited then the alkalosis persists.

(b) **False** Hyperventilation causes a respiratory alkalosis.

(c) **True** The functioning kidney excretes 'fixed' acids.

(d) **True** Ketoacids are formed by incomplete degradation of fatty acids.

(e) **False** Potassium and hydrogen ions compete for exchange with sodium ions in the renal tubule and at cell membranes. A low extracellular potassium concentration leads to increased passage of hydrogen ions into the urine and into cells.

68 (a) **True** The portion of the saline remaining in the circulation will dilute the red blood cells.

(b) **False** Dilution of the plasma proteins allows much of the fluid to pass into the interstitial space. Saline, therefore, has limited value in treating blood loss.

(c) **True** Surgery increases secretion of aldosterone and antidiuretic hormone (ADH).

(d) **False** Water dilutes the blood fluids and the reduced osmolarity lowers ADH secretion.Water is therefore rapidly eliminated in the urine. Saline does not reduce osmolarity of the body fluids and ADH secretion is not suppressed. Slower mechanisms such as reducing aldosterone secretion and raising levels of atrial natriuretic factor are required.

(e) **True** The raised central nervous pressure stimulates via the atrial receptors vasodilatation in skeletal muscle.

69 In man, renal clearance of
   (a) glucose is normally zero.
   (b) sodium is increased by aldosterone.
   (c) creatinine is half of normal in a person who had a unilateral nephrectomy one
       year previously.
   (d) para-aminohippurate measures renal blood flow.
   (e) free water occurs only when the urine is hypotonic compared to plasma.

70 The urinary bladder
   (a) cannot empty when it contains less than 100 ml.
   (b) pressure rises linearly as the volume increases.
   (c) stretch receptors contain intrafusal muscle fibres.
   (d) will be emptied within one hour after drinking one litre of water.
   (e) is mainly innervated by the lumbar segments of the spinal cord.

69 (a) **True**   No glucose appears in urine until plasma glucose concentration exeeds 10 mM (180 mg 100 ml^{-1}).

(b) **False**   Aldosterone reduces sodium excretion.

(c) **False**   Compensatory hypertrophy occurs in the remaining kidney and glomerular filtration rate exceeds 50% of normal.

(d) **False**   It measures the plasma flow through the kidney.

(e) **True** C_{H_2O} = urine volume − C_{OSM}.

If urine is hypertonic, then C_{OSM} > urine volume.

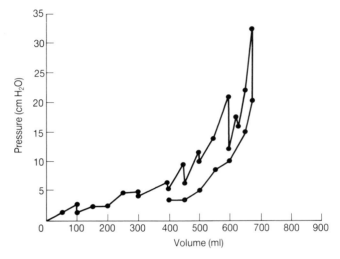

Fig. 2.2 Cystometrogram. Changes of pressure in the human bladder during filling and emptying. Water was run slowly into the bladder and the pressure measured after each 50 ml. It was then allowed to slowly empty.

70 (a) **False**   Voluntary straining may empty the bladder when it contains only 10–20 ml.

(b) **False**   See Fig. 2.2.

(c) **False**   The bladder is composed of smooth muscle and the stretch receptors are not muscle spindles.

(d) **True**   Drinking large volumes of water induces a marked diuresis, producing at least 400 ml in an hour – a volume which will initiate the desire to micturate.

(e) **False**   Both sensory and motor nerves come from the sacral segments of the cord.

EAST GLAMORGAN GENERAL HOSPITAL LIBRARY

CHURCH VILLAGE, near PONTYPRIDD

71 Angiotensin II
   (a) is the only stimulator of aldosterone release.
   (b) causes vasoconstriction.
   (c) is formed as blood passes through the lungs.
   (d) stimulates the sensation of thirst.
   (e) levels in the plasma are increased by sympathetic nerve stimulation to the kidney.

72 Gastric acid secretion
   (a) can be stimulated by an injection of insulin.
   (b) is increased following removal of the pyloric antrum.
   (c) is inhibited by histamine (H_2)-blocking drugs.
   (d) has no effect on gastric emptying.
   (e) is reduced by antacids.

73 Nitrogen balance in the acute surgical patient
   (a) is more negative following severe burns than after major elective surgery.
   (b) in the catabolic phase is associated with positive potassium balance.
   (c) can be completely corrected by administering 2000 Kcal day^{-1}
   (d) reflects increased protein turnover with synthesis exceeding breakdown.
   (e) is entirely due to the gluconeogenic effect of cortisol.

74. A subject weighing 70 kg who at rest is using 250 ml min^{-1} O_2 and producing 200 ml min^{-1} CO_2:
   (a) has a respiratory exchange ratio (R) of 1.250.
   (b) has been deprived of food for 3 days.
   (c) is hyperthyroid.
   (d) is using both fat and carbohydrate for oxidative metabolism.
   (e) was hyperventilating during the measurement of gas exchange.

75 A negative nitrogen balance occurs
   (a) during puberty.
   (b) when vomiting is prolonged.
   (c) during weight training.
   (d) in the early puerperium.
   (e) when protein intake is 5 g day^{-1}.

71 (a) **False**   Aldosterone is also released by ACTH and by raised levels of circulating potassium.

(b) **True**   By a direct action in arterioles. It also raises blood pressure by a central action.

(c) **True**   High levels of converting enzyme are located in the endothelial cells of the pulmonary vascular bed.

(d) **True**   By acting on circumventricular organs which are outside the blood–brain barrier.

(e) **True**   Stimulation of sympathetic nerves to the kidney increases secretion of renin.

72 (a) **True**   This is the basis of Hollander's test of vagal integrity. An intravenous injection of insulin lowers the blood glucose concentration, which stimulates acid secretion through a medullary centre and the vagus nerve.

(b) **False**   The antrum secretes gastrin which is one of the main stimulators of acid secretion from the body and fundus of the stomach.

(c) **True**   Histamine is a transmitter in the stimulation of acid secretion. Drugs such as cimetidine are important in the treatment of peptic ulceration.

(d) **False**   Highly acid gastric contents entering the duodenum reflexly inhibit emptying of the stomach.

(e) **False**   Antacids, by neutralizing the acid, may increase the rate of secretion.

73 (a) **True**   This may reflect the large amount of protein damaged by heat and plasma protein exuded through damaged capillaries.

(b) **False**   Protein breakdown is associated with loss of intracellular fluid and hence of potassium.

(c) **False**   Adequate calorie nutrition reduces the negative nitrogen balance but does not completely prevent it.

(d) **False**   Breakdown exceeds synthesis.

(e) **False**   Cortisol is only one factor.

74 (a) **False** $$R = \frac{VCO_2}{VO_2} = 0.800$$

(b) **False**   The subject would be metabolizing mainly fat and R would be nearer 0.7.

(c) **False**   This is a normal oxygen consumption for a subject of this size.

(d) **True**   When using carbohydrate for metabolism R is 1.0; when metabolising fat it is 0.7.

(e) **False**   During hyperventilation R rises towards, and may exceed, 1.0.

75 (a) **False**   This is a period of rapid growth and nitrogen balance will be positive.

(b) **True**   No protein is entering the body and there may be actual loss in the gastric juice.

(c) **False**   Weight training increases the mass of muscle.

(d) **True**   Losses occur due to the lochia, the involution of the uterus and reduction of plasma volume.

(e) **True**   The minimum requirement for a person to remain in nitrogen balance is probably 40 g day^{-1} of protein in the diet.

76 The duodenum
    (a) controls the secretion of bile.
    (b) can slow gastric emptying.
    (c) absorbs no nutrients.
    (d) controls the volume but not the enzyme content of pancreatic juice.
    (e) absorbs vitamin B_{12}.

77 The large intestine
    (a) receives at least one litre of fluid per day through the ileocaecal valve.
    (b) contains bacteria that synthesize vitamin K.
    (c) can secrete K^+ ions into its lumen.
    (d) is stimulated by gastrin to produce mass movements.
    (e) contents produce ammonia.

78 Bilirubin glucuronide
    (a) in obstructive jaundice is excreted in the urine.
    (b) is produced in the spleen.
    (c) is concentrated in the gall bladder.
    (d) production will be reduced in haemolytic anaemia.
    (e) is the main brown pigment in the faeces.

79 Malabsorption of fat from the gastrointestinal tract
    (a) may reduce the coagulability of blood.
    (b) is always due to obstruction of the bile duct or the pancreatic duct.
    (c) is likely following resection of the terminal ileum.
    (d) ensures that no fat is layed down in adipose tissue.
    (e) may cause defects of cell membranes.

76 (a) **False**   Cholecystokin/pancreozymin (CCK/PZ) controls release of bile from the gall bladder but **not** secretion of bile by the liver.

  (b) **True**   Hypertonic fluid, high-fat levels and high acidity in the duodenum slow the rate of gastric emptying.

  (c) **False**   Many nutrients, provided they are suitably digested, can be absorbed from the duodenum.

  (d) **False**   Secretin stimulates the main volume components and CCK/PZ the enzyme content.

  (e) **False**   Vitamin B_{12} is only absorbed in the terminal ileum.

77 (a) **True**   About 1.5 litres of fluid pass each day into the colon. Approximately 1.3 litres are absorbed and 0.2 litres are passed in the faeces.

  (b) **True**   A significant proportion of the body's requirements for vitamin K may be synthesized in the lumen of the colon.

  (c) **True**   When K^+ intake is high, aldosterone increases sodium coupled secretion of K^+ into the lumen of the colon.

  (d) **True**   This is the gastrocolic reflex, and accounts for the frequency with which defaecation follows a meal.

  (e) **True**   Ammonia produced by bacteria is absorbed into the portal circulation and detoxicated in the liver.

78 (a) **True**   Bilirubin glucuronide is soluble and can be filtered through the glomerulus.

  (b) **False**   Bilirubin is produced in the spleen (and elsewhere in the reticuloendothelial system) and conjugated with glucuronic acid in the liver.

  (c) **True**   It may be concentrated up to ten times.

  (d) **False**   Increased red cell breakdown results in increased quantities of bilirubin, which are conjugated in the liver.

  (e) **False**   In the gastrointestinal tract bilirubin is converted to stercobilinogen and stercobilin. The latter is responsible for the brown colour of faeces.

79 (a) **True**   Absorption of fat-soluble vitamin K is impaired and this will reduce the synthesis of clotting factors, especially prothrombin.

  (b) **False**   It could be due to pathology of the intestine.

  (c) **True**   The bile salts are reabsorbed in this region and their enterohepatic circulation will be impaired.

  (d) **False**   If excess calories are present in the body, fatty acids can be synthesized from glucose.

  (e) **True**   There are some essential fatty acids. Deficiency results in defects of the cell wall.

80 Swallowing
   (a) depends on the integrity of the vagus nerves.
   (b) may move solids and liquids against gravity.
   (c) is blocked by atropine.
   (d) inhibits ventilation.
   (e) must be prevented during estimation of intrapleural pressure with a balloon
       in the oesophagus.

81 Noradrenaline
   (a) is the sympathetic neurotransmitter at α-adrenoceptors but not at β-
       adrenoceptors.
   (b) constricts blood vessels in skeletal muscle.
   (c) when infused intravenously slows heart rate.
   (d) increases metabolic rate in human babies.
   (e) induced vasoconstriction in the skin may be blocked by propranolol.

82 Insulin secretion may be increased
   (a) following a meal.
   (b) by hypersecretion of growth hormone.
   (c) during an infection.
   (d) during exercise.
   (e) during pregnancy.

83 Conduction of an impulse through a nervous pathway
   (a) increases in velocity as it spreads away from the cell body.
   (b) can pass both ways across a synapse.
   (c) slows at each synapse.
   (d) depends on the presence of extracellular sodium ions.
   (e) speeds up as temperature increases.

80 (a) **True** The vagus innervates the muscles of the pharynx and oesophagus.

  (b) **True** Swallowing can successfully occur in subjects tilted head down or doing handstands.

  (c) **False** The muscles involved are striated. The neuromuscular junction could be blocked with a muscle relaxant.

  (d) **True** Ventilation ceases during swallowing, otherwise food and liquids would be aspirated into the respiratory tract.

  (e) **True** Measurement of intrapleural pressure with an oesophageal balloon depends on closure of the upper and lower oesophagus and the absence of peristaltic waves.

81 (a) **False** The sympathetic neurotransmitter at all adrenergic sites is noradrenaline. Circulating adrenaline may have a relatively greater effect on β-adrenoceptors.

  (b) **True** The muscle vascular bed is large and is involved in blood pressure homeostasis. Exercise-induced vasodilatation and vasodilatation as part of the defence reaction are due to separate mechanisms.

  (c) **True** The strong α effect raises blood pressure by peripheral vasoconstriction. The heart rate is then slowed by the baroreceptor reflex acting through the vagus nerve.

  (d) **True** The sympathetic system activates brown adipose tissue in babies.

  (e) **False** Vasoconstriction is an α-adrenoceptor action and cannot be blocked by a β-antagonist

82 (a) **True** Plasma glucose concentration rises and directly stimulates insulin release. Preabsorption, there may be stimulation of the islets by hormones from the gastrointestinal tract.

  (b) **True** High levels of growth hormone raise plasma glucose concentration.

  (c) **True** Insulin requirements are increased by infections.

  (d) **False** Increased utilization of glucose facilitates its uptake by cells and the insulin requirement falls.

  (e) **True** The greater mass of maternal and foetal tissues increases insulin requirements.

83 (a) **False** Conduction in a fibre is slower in the more peripheral regions.

  (b) **False** Antidromic conduction can occur in a nerve fibre but **not** across a synapse.

  (c) **True** There is a finite delay at a synapse.

  (d) **True** Depolarization of the nerve fibre to provide the action potential requires influx of sodium ions.

  (e) **True** Like most biological phenomena, nerve conduction velocity increases with temperature.

84 Chronic administration of glucocorticoids at levels in excess of normal rates of
   secretion will increase the likelihood of
   (a) developing diabetes mellitus.
   (b) impaired healing of wounds.
   (c) hypertrophy of the adrenal cortex.
   (d) death following trauma.
   (e) suppression of the immune response.

85 Following hypophysectomy
   (a) there is persistent diabetes insipidus.
   (b) sodium loss in the urine is high.
   (c) thyroxine should be given to prevent hypothyroidism.
   (d) hypoglycaemia is more likely to occur.
   (e) in a 30-year-old woman, menstruation will continue normally.

86 The stretch reflex
   (a) is initiated in the muscle spindles.
   (b) is polysynaptic.
   (c) inhibits the antagonist muscle(s).
   (d) is absent when there is a spastic paralysis if the limb.
   (e) activates the Renshaw cell.

84 (a) **True**   Excess glucocorticoids increase gluconeogenesis and inhibit glucose uptake by tissues, thereby increasing blood glucose concentration and raising insulin requirements.

   (b) **True**   May reflect their action on body protein.

   (c) **False**   ACTH release is suppressed and the adrenals atrophy.

   (d) **True**   Survival of stresses such as trauma requires an increased secretion of cortisol, which cannot be achieved when the adrenals have atrophied.

   (e) **True**   Steroids are used clinically to suppress immune responses, e.g. to prevent rejection of transplants.

85 (a) **False**   Vasopressin is produced by neurones in the supraoptic nucleus and, after healing of the stalk, secretion into the blood can again occur.

   (b) **False**   Aldosterone secretion does not depend upon ACTH.

   (c) **True**   Thyroxine secretion is very low in the absence of TSH.

   (d) **True**   Two mechanisms for raising blood glucose concentration in an emergency have been eliminated, i.e. growth hormone and ACTH/cortisol.

   (e) **False**   Cyclical ovarian function depends upon circulating FSH and LH.

86 (a) **True**   See (a) in Fig. 2.3.

   (b) **False**   Measurement of the reflex latency suggests that there can be only one synapse.

   (c) **True**   By a polysynaptic pathway so that antagonists relax slightly after agonists begin to contract.

   (d) **False**   Reflexes are potentiated by an upper motor neurone lesion.

   (e) **True**   The Renshaw loop, (e) in Fig. 2.3, is a mechanism for self limiting the reflex.

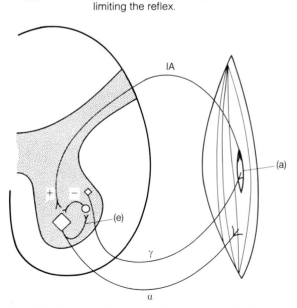

Fig. 2.3 The stretch reflex pathway. α α-motorneurone; γ fusimotor neurone; 1A afferent fibre from primary afferent in spindle; (a) muscle spindle; (e) Renshaw cell and loop.

87 Cerebrospinal fluid
  (a) is produced at a rate not exceeding 100 ml day^{-1}.
  (b) composition indicates that it cannot be formed by active secretion.
  (c) flows from the third to the fourth ventricle.
  (d) is formed only in the choroid plexi.
  (e) drains into cerebral lymphatics.

88 With reference to the organs of special sense,
  (a) the near point for vision lengthens with age.
  (b) low frequency sounds stimulate units towards the apex of cochlea.
  (c) the sensation of bitterness is recognized near the back of the tongue.
  (d) a person who is spun to his left in a rotating chair, develops the sensation of spinning to his right when the chair is suddenly stopped.
  (e) colour vision is a function of the rods in the retina.

87 (a) **False** The normal rate of production is 400–500 ml day^{-1}.

(b) **False** Some components have a lower concentration in CSF than in plasma (e.g. potassium, glucose) whilst others have a higher concentration (e.g. magnesium, chloride).

(c) **True** CSF is formed in the mainly choroid plexi of the lateral ventricles and flows into the third ventricle and then through the aquaduct into the fourth ventricle. It then leaves the fourth ventricle via its dorsal foramina to enter the subarachnoid space.

(d) **False** Fluid also flows across the ependyma lining the ventricles and across the arachnoid membrane.

(e) **False** There are no lymphatics in the CNS; drainage is via the arachnoid granulations into the venous sinuses.

88 (a) **True** With increasing age most people with previously normal sight require spectacles for reading because they are unable to accommodate.

(b) **True** Low-frequency sounds stimulate units towards the apex whilst high-frequency sounds stimulate those nearer to the oval window.

(c) **True** Other sensations are appreciated further forward on the tongue.

(d) **True** When spinning begins, the head spins faster than the fluid in the semi-circular canals and the subject feels he is going in the direction of spin. When the head suddenly stops, the fluid continues to spin, giving the sensation of reversal of direction.

(e) **False** Colour vision is a function of the cones.

89 Pain
  (a) impulses are conducted to the spinal cord only in unmyelinated fibres.
  (b) due to carcinoma of the pancreas, may be relieved by ablation of the coeliac (sympathetic) ganglion.
  (c) intensity may be lessened by simultaneous stimulation of touch receptors of the same segments.
  (d) relief achieved by section of a peripheral nerve may subsequently become worsened.
  (e) in a phantom limb is less likely if good analgesia is achieved in the limb pre-amputation.

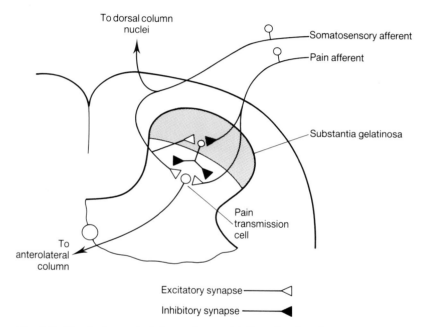

Fig. 2.4 The 'gate control' theory for modulation of pain afferents. If the pain afferent activates the transmission cell, pain will be felt. However, if large sensory afferents are also stimulated, these activate an interneurone in the substantia gelatinosa, which presynaptically inhibits all input to the pain transmission cell.

90 Following complete transection of the spinal cord at the C6–7 level
  (a) vital capacity is reduced by over 50%.
  (b) the heart will not be slowed by an increase in arterial blood pressure.
  (c) sweating is not abolished on the face.
  (d) reflexes in segments below the lesion will reappear in the lowest segments first.
  (e) reflex emptying of the bladder occurs within 24 hours.

89 (a) **False** Pain impulses are conducted by myelinated A-δ and in unmyelinated C fibres.

(b) **True** Fibres from visceral pain receptors run with the sympathetic nerves before entering the cord via the white ramus communicans and the posterior root.

(c) **True** This is the basis of gating (see Fig. 2.4).

(d) **True** Neuromas may form at the proximal cut end of the nerve trunk and axons regrowing from pain fibres may fire spontaneously.

(e) **True** It is important to achieve analgesia either by systemic drugs or with local anaesthetic block prior to amputation, otherwise the patient may continue to experience pain which he perceives to arise in the missing limb.

90 (a) **True** There is no intercostal breathing but the phrenic nerves are still supplied by the respiratory centre and so diaphragmatic breathing can occur.

(b) **False** Afferents from the baroreceptors will be intact and the heart can be slowed by impulses in the vagus nerve.

(c) **False** There are no connections between the hypothalamus and the and the highest outflow (T1) of the sympathetic system.

(d) **True** The earliest reflexes to reappear are those of the sacral segments.

(e) **False** The bladder fills until overflow incontinence occurs. Careful treatment with early catheterization and regular emptying of the bladder is needed if reflex micturition is eventually to be established.

91 The calcium content of bone is increased by
   (a) prolonged bedrest.
   (b) increased secretion of parathyroid hormone.
   (c) administration of oestrogens to post-menopausal women.
   (d) prolonged administration of glucocorticoids.
   (e) a successful kidney transplant to a patient in renal failure.

92 In the deeply anaesthetized patient undergoing abdominal surgery
   (a) sweating does not occur in a warm environment because of premedication with atropine.
   (b) heat loss will be reduced when the abdomen is opened.
   (c) hypothermia will persist for the first 3 days of recovery.
   (d) shivering will occur if the theatre is cold.
   (e) heat production will be increased for a few days after operation.

93 From the late teens to the 60s
   (a) diastolic arterial blood pressure decreases.
   (b) plasma sodium concentration increases.
   (c) basal metabolic rate decreases.
   (d) cardiac output at rest increases.
   (e) residual volume of the lungs increases.

94 During a period of dynamic exercise
   (a) plasma volume increases.
   (b) heart rate increases relatively more than stroke volume.
   (c) P_ACO_2 does not change from the resting level until the work load is moderately severe.
   (d) there is an oxygen debt even if lactate is not produced.
   (e) splanchnic blood flow is reduced.

95 The sudden loss of **one** litre of blood from the body will
   (a) lower central venous pressure.
   (b) reduce excretion of sodium in the urine.
   (c) raise the concentration of lactate in the plasma.
   (d) increase vagal tone to the heart.
   (e) not immediately reduce the haemoglobin concentration.

91 (a) **False** Inactivity and reduced exposure to gravity lead to removal of calcium from bone.

(b) **False** Parathyroid hormone removes calcium from bone.

(c) **True** Sex hormones have an anabolic action and this is now a common treatment.

(d) **False** Glucocorticoids have a catabolic effect on proteins, including those in bone. Removal of bone proteins leads to osteoporosis.

(e) **True** The functioning kidney converts vitamin D to the active form 1,25-dihydroxycholecalciferol. This increases absorption of calcium from the intestine and increases uptake into bone.

92 (a) **True** Atropine blocks the cholinergic receptors in sweat glands.

(b) **False** Evaporative heat loss readily occurs from the peritoneum.

(c) **False** There is usually a sterile pyrexia following surgery probably caused by tissue breakdown products acting as pyrogens.

(d) **False** Deep anaesthesia blocks the shivering mechanisms centrally, and muscle relaxant drugs block the neuromuscular junction.

(e) **True** This is part of the metabolic response to trauma.

93 (a) **False** In males diastolic pressure steadily increases with age; in females it changes little until the menopause when a steady increase begins.

(b) **False** There are no age-related changes.

(c) **True** In males, basal metabolic rate falls from 175 kJ m^{-2} $hour^{-1}$ aged 20 to 146 kJ m^{-2} $hour^{-1}$ aged 65.

(d) **False** May parallel the decrease in basal metabolic rate.

(e) **True** The chest wall stiffens so that forced expiration cannot empty the chest to the same extent.

94 (a) **False** Fluid is lost from the plasma into active muscle and packed cell volume increases.

(b) **True** Heart rate may increase 2.5–3 times (e.g. 65–180 beats per minute), whilst stroke volume seldom doubles (e.g. 70–120 ml).

(c) **True** In mild to moderate exercise, ventilation is appropriate for the increased gas exchange and P_ACO_2 is unchanged. Above 60% VO_2 max, increasing levels of lactic acid additionally stimulates ventilation, and P_ACO_2 falls.

(d) **True** At the beginning of exercise, the oxygen used by tissues exceeds that entering at the lungs, and oxygen is provided from the stores, particularly that in the venous blood.

(e) **True** There are marked reductions in flow to the gastrointestinal tract and to the liver.

95 (a) **True** Reduction of volume will be more evident in the venous compartment.

(b) **True** Aldosterone secretion is increased; ANF level is reduced.

(c) **True** Tissues made ischaemic by intense vasoconstriction may metabolize anaerobically.

(d) **False** Vagal tone is reduced by the baroreceptor reflex contributing to the increase of heart rate.

(e) **True** The remaining blood is only slowly diluted with fluid moving across the capillaries from the interstitial space.

96 During a long period of bedrest
  (a) basal heart rate increases.
  (b) excretion of calcium in the urine is reduced.
  (c) plasma volume increases.
  (d) orthostatic intolerance develops.
  (e) there is a reduction of urinary excretion of vannilyl-mandelic acid (VMA).

97 During a normal pregnancy
  (a) skin bloodflow of the mother is increased.
  (b) maternal plasma volume increases.
  (c) the ureters of the mother dilate.
  (d) plasma cortisol concentration rises in the mother.
  (e) foetal haemoglobin concentration exceeds 20 g dl^{-1}.

98 During puberty
  (a) in the female, breast enlargement precedes the appearance of pubic hair.
  (b) ovulation precedes the menarché bleed.
  (c) the levels of oestrogen or testosterone required to suppress gonadotrophin secretion are increased.
  (d) elevation of the secretion of oestrogens precedes that of progesterone by some months.
  (e) enlargement of the testes precedes growth of the accessory sex organs.

99 A normal man weighing 70 kg sitting quietly at rest
  (a) is losing less than 10% of his heat production by evaporation.
  (b) is producing more than 3 Kcal (12 kJ) heat per minute.
  (c) is manufacturing between 15 and 30 ml red blood cells per day.
  (d) is deriving over 10% of his energy expenditure from amino acids.
  (e) has a cardiac oxygen consumption between 20 and 30 ml min^{-1}.

96 (a) **True** The heart becomes detrained.
   (b) **False** Reduced exposure to gravitational forces and to the stresses of muscle contraction increases calcium loss from bone.
   (c) **False** Central blood volume is raised when lying and this leads to natriuresis and diuresis and an overall reduction of plasma volume.
   (d) **True** Normally blood pressure is little affected by standing, but following only a few days bedrest marked falls in blood pressure occur on standing.
   (e) **True** Reduced exercise and postural adaptation lower the activity of the sympathetic system.

97 (a) **True** The increased tissue volume of the mother and the foetus increase heat production. Vasodilatation in the skin increases heat loss.
   (b) **True** This may reflect the increasing volume of the vascular bed.
   (c) **True** Progesterone relaxes smooth muscle.
   (d) **True** Oestrogens increase production of cortisol-binding globulin in the liver. This reduces the concentration of free cortisol, and secretion of cortisol increases to give a normal level of free hormone in the plasma.
   (e) **True** High haemoglobin concentration is necessary to transport oxygen at low PO_2.

98 (a) **True** In most girls the major events of puberty occur in the order: breast development, appearance of pubic hair, menarché.
   (b) **False** The first few cycles are anovulatory.
   (c) **True** An important factor in raising gonadotrophin secretion is the reduced feedback effects of gonadal hormones.
   (d) **False** Progesterone appears in significant quantities only when ovulation occurs and a corpus luteum is formed.
   (e) **True** Enlargement of accessory sex organs depends on elevated levels of testosterone.

99 (a) **False** Evaporative water loss through the skin and in the breath is at least 1200 ml day^{-1} or 50 ml hour^{-1}. Since one litre of water by evaporation removes 2400 kJ from the body, about 100 kJ hour^{-1} are lost by this route. Resting metabolic rate is about 300 kJ hour^{-1}.
   (b) **False** Resting metabolic rate is about 5 kJ minute^{-1}.
   (c) **True** Red blood cells persist for about 100 days, so that 1% turn over each day. Total red cell volume is about 2000 ml, therefore about 20 ml are renewed each day.
   (d) **True** When the body is in protein balance, an amount of protein equal to the intake is deaminated and metabolized. A daily intake of protein of 70 g will yield about 60 g of carbon skeleton, which in turn will produce about 1000 kJ energy.
   (e) **True** The myocardium utilizes about 10% of the total oxygen consumption, i.e., about 25 ml minute^{-1}.

100 Following major surgery to the gastrointestinal tract, at the stage when no fluid can be given by mouth
- (a) the patient's energy requirements can be met by infusion of isotonic glucose solution.
- (b) the patient's fluid balance can be maintained by infusion of 3 litres of isotonic saline solution per day.
- (c) fluid aspirated from the stomach will be hypertonic.
- (d) potassium supplements should be injected directly into the intravenous catheter.
- (e) fluid volumes should be adjusted to give urine production of at least one litre per day.

100 (a) **False** One litre 5% glucose is equivalent to only 200 Kcal or 840 kJ.

(b) **False** Following surgery patients retain sodium, so this fluid would largely remain in the body, leading to circulatory overload and oedema.

(c) **False** Most gastrointestinal secretions are isotonic and saliva is hypotonic.

(d) **False** Injection of isotonic potassium chloride as a bolus will give a transiently high potassium concentration in the plasma, which will be toxic to the heart. KCl should be diluted by adding it to the infusion bag.

(e) **True** Normal urine volume is at least **one** litre a day.

3 Pathology

101 In chronic iron deficiency anaemia there is characteristically
   (a) an atrophic gastritis.
   (b) a low mean corpuscular haemoglobin.
   (c) a low mean corpuscular volume (MCV).
   (d) a reduced total iron-binding capacity.
   (e) megaloblastic changes in the bone marrow.

102 Sickle cell disease gives rise to
   (a) increased susceptibility to infections with encapsulated organisms.
   (b) a haemolytic anaemia.
   (c) an amino-acid substitution on the haem molecule.
   (d) an elevated reticulocyte count.
   (e) an increased susceptibility to *P. falciparum*.

103 The following are recognized complications of blood transfusion
   (a) hepatitis C.
   (b) haemosiderosis.
   (c) hyperkalaemia.
   (d) ABO incompatibity when group A blood is given to an AB recipient.
   (e) cytomegalovirus infection.

104 In the investigation of a bleeding disorder
   (a) the prothrombin time ratio is usually raised in haemophilia A.
   (b) liver failure decreases factor VIII production.
   (c) an increased bleeding time suggests a platelet abnormality.
   (d) disseminated intravascular coagulation is usually associated with a decreased platelet count.
   (e) severe thrombocytopenia causes an abnormal partial thromboplastin time.

105 A raised count of neutrophil polymorphonuclear leucocytes in the peripheral blood is usually seen with
   (a) diabetes mellitus.
   (b) chronic granulocytic leukaemia.
   (c) intraduct carcinoma of the breast.
   (d) acute hepatitis due to hepatitis A.
   (e) acute salpingitis.

101 (a) **False** This is seen in pernicious anaemia.
   (b) **True** The red cells are characteristically hypochromic.
   (c) **True** The red cells are characteristically microcytic.
   (d) **False** It is characteristically raised.
   (e) **False** The red cell precursors are normoblastic in iron deficiency anaemia.

102 (a) **True** Particularly *Strep. pneumoniae*. In some countries, typhoid osteo-myelitis results from infection of bone infarcts.
   (b) **True** There is a decreased red cell survival.
   (c) **False** Haemoglobin S shows valine substituted for glutamic acid at position 6 on the beta chain of the globin molecule.
   (d) **True** Indicates young red cells in peripheral blood.
   (e) **False** There is a relative resistance to *P. falciparum* though patients still die of this infection.

103 (a) **True** It is responsible for many of the non-A, non-B post-transfusion hepatitis cases.
   (b) **True** Where many transfusions are given in conditions such as chronic anaemias.
   (c) **True** Uncommon but may be a problem with old blood, with neonates and with patients in renal failure.
   (d) **False** The recipient would not have anti A in his plasma.
   (e) **True** May be a serious problem in immunosuppressed recipients.

104 (a) **False** It is normal: factor VIII does not influence the prothrombin time.
   (b) **False** The liver is not the source of factor VIII.
   (c) **True** Though vessel wall abnormalities may increase the bleeding time, platelet abnormalities are more common.
   (d) **True** There is a consumption coagulopathy that involves coagulation factors including platelets.
   (e) **False** The patient's platelets are not involved in the partial thrombo-plastin time.

105 (a) **False** Not unless a complication occurs which causes a neutrophilia.
   (b) **True** Neutrophil granulocytes are raised in the peripheral blood.
   (c) **False** Usually there are no significant changes in the blood picture.
   (d) **False** Lymphocytes are increased in the liver and may also be raised in peripheral blood.
   (e) **True** Usually caused by a pyogenic organism.

106 The following cells belong to the mononuclear phagocyte system
    (a) epithelioid cells.
    (b) neutrophil polymorphonuclear leucocytes.
    (c) Langhans' type giant cells.
    (d) eosinophils.
    (e) macrophages.

107 The major histocompatibility complex (MHC) encodes for
    (a) haemophilia A.
    (b) class I HLA molecules.
    (c) class II HLA molecules.
    (d) the ABO blood group system.
    (e) some complement components.

108 The following diseases have a well-recognized association with particular HLA antigens
    (a) familial polyposis coli.
    (b) insulin-dependent diabetes.
    (c) Cushing's disease.
    (d) coeliac disease.
    (e) haemochromatosis.

109 Type I (anaphylactic type) hypersensitivity reactions
    (a) usually occur in people with a history of allergy.
    (b) cause relaxation of smooth muscle in pulmonary vessels.
    (c) are characteristically mediated via mast cell degranulation.
    (d) characteristically involve IgA at mucosal surfaces.
    (e) are partly mediated by leukotrienes.

110 Formation of immune type giant cell granulomas in tissue
    (a) requires involvement of T-helper cells.
    (b) is characteristic of renal transplant rejection.
    (c) requires the presence of blood-derived monocytes.
    (d) is diagnostic of tuberculosis.
    (e) is often seen in temporal arteritis.

106 (a) **True** In immune granulomas macrophages may develop prominent eosinophilic cytoplasm giving them an 'epithelioid' appearance (ultrastructurally the rough endoplasmic reticulum and Golgi have become more developed).

(b) **False** These cells are short-lived phagocytes and are members of the granulocyte cell series.

(c) **True** Fusion of macrophages in granulomas may give rise to these multinucleate cells.

(d) **False** These belong to the granulocyte series.

(e) **True** Monocytes in the blood stream migrate into the tissues and become actively phagocytic macrophages.

107 (a) **False** The MHC is on chromosome 6. Haemophilia A is X-linked.

(b) **True** Coded by three loci HLA-A, HLA-B and HLA-C.

(c) **True** Coded by locus HLA-D and are less widely distributed than class I.

(d) **False** Class I HLA molecules are found on nucleated cells, not red cells.

(e) **True** C2 and C4 are coded in the MHC and, with other molecules, are grouped as Class III MHC molecules.

108 (a) **False** It is not HLA-linked.

(b) **True** DR3, DR4.

(c) **False** It is not HLA-linked.

(d) **True** B8, DR3, DR7.

(e) **True** A3.

109 (a) **True** But they may occur without such a history.

(b) **False** The pulmonary arterioles tend to be constricted when the lung is involved.

(c) **True** Antigen unites with antibody, usually IgE, which has previously fixed to the mast-cell membrane.

(d) **False** Typically IgE is involved.

(e) **True** B4, C4, D4, E4.

110 (a) **True** CD4-positive cells are required for sensitization and subsequent release of lymphokines, which influence the macrophages that predominate in the granuloma.

(b) **False** Though cell-mediated reactions are often involved they usually involve T cell-mediated cytotoxicity rather than granuloma formation.

(c) **True** Monocytes are recruited and become macrophages in the tissue. Epithelioid cells and multinucleate giant cells (macrophage polykaryons) are subsequently derived from them.

(d) **False** Granulomas develop in many diseases.

(e) **True** Giant cell granulomas develop, associated with damaged elastica (hence the term giant cell arteritis).

111 In acute inflammation the following factors increase the permeability of small blood vessels
    (a) leukotrienes.
    (b) interleukin I.
    (c) bradykinin.
    (d) histamine.
    (e) C5a.

112 The following are frequently found in pus
    (a) histiocytes.
    (b) dead bacteria.
    (c) live bacteria.
    (d) plasma cells.
    (e) eosinophils.

113 Granulation tissue formation
    (a) does not usually occur in T cell-deficient patients.
    (b) is usually accompanied by the presence of multinucleate giant cells (macrophage polykaryons).
    (c) delays wound healing.
    (d) is usually followed by fibrosis.
    (e) characteristically shows angioneogenesis.

114 Cells of the following lines may regenerate well after some have been destroyed
    (a) posterior root ganglion cells.
    (b) renal proximal convoluted tubular cells.
    (c) hepatocytes.
    (d) chondrocytes of hyaline cartilage.
    (e) mucus-secreting cells of the gastric mucosa.

115 In the healing of a closed fracture of a long bone
    (a) the presence of devitalized bone delays healing.
    (b) provisional callus formation is delayed if granulation tissue forms.
    (c) woven bone formation indicates ischaemia at the site of fracture.
    (d) bony callus is formed by endochondral and subperiosteal ossification.
    (e) infection at the site accelerates bony union.

116 In the healing of a large open wound caused by trauma
    (a) skin adnexae do not regenerate.
    (b) Vitamin A deficiency delays collagen maturation.
    (c) contraction of the wound is brought about by the shortening of collagen fibres.
    (d) plasma cells are the predominant inflammatory cell in the connective tissue.
    (e) platelet-derived growth factor stimulates mitosis in squamous epithelial cells.

111 (a) **True**   Partly responsible for the delayed sustained increase in permeability.

    (b) **False**   Main effects in acute inflammation are on endothelium.

    (c) **True**   Activated Hageman factor acts on kininogen in plasma to give the very short-lived bradykinin.

    (d) **True**   Quickly released from mast cells and is largely responsible for the immediate short-lived increase in permeability.

    (e) **True**   Following complement activation C5 convertase breaks off C5a, which is chemotactic for polymorphs and increases vascular permeability.

112 (a) **True**   These are seen in the 'demolition' phase of acute inflammation and, as macrophages, in pus.

    (b) **True**   These are frequently present.

    (c) **True**   They can often be cultured from pus.

    (d) **False**   They are uncommonly seen.

    (e) **False**   They are uncommonly seen. The most common cell in pus is the neutrophil polymorphonuclear leucocyte ('neutrophils', 'polys' or 'pus cells').

113 (a) **False**   It is not dependant on the specific immune response.

    (b) **False**   They may, however, be seen occasionally.

    (c) **False**   It is required for wound healing.

    (d) **True**   Organization by granulation tissue usually results in fibrosis.

    (e) **True**   New capillary formation is an essential part of granulation tissue.

114 (a) **False**   Ganglion cells are post-mitotic cells and do not regenerate. Axons may be reconstituted only if the ganglion cell is viable.

    (b) **True**   This happens after acute tubular necrosis, provided the cause has been removed.

    (c) **True**   Hepatocytes have a well-developed regenerative capacity.

    (d) **False**   Though capable of some regeneration it is usually very limited.

    (e) **True**   Epithelial surfaces can usually regenerate well.

115 (a) **True**   This has to be metabolized before healing is completed.

    (b) **False**   Granulation tissue is an essential part of the formation of provisional callus.

    (c) **False**   Woven bone usually forms first before remodelling into lamellar bone.

    (d) **True**   The cartilage islands, which form in granulation tissue, ossify by the endochondral process.

    (e) **False**   Infection has to be eliminated before bony union is complete.

116 (a) **True**   Residual adnexae may, however, act as a source of new squamous cells when a wound (or burn) is not full thickness.

    (b) **False**   Vitamin A has its effects on the epithelium in wound healing.

    (c) **False**   It probably results from the action of myofibroblasts.

    (d) **False**   Histiocytes usually predominate.

    (e) **False**   Epidermal growth factor stimulates growth of epithelial cells.

117 The following factors increase the risk of postoperative pneumonia
    (a) pulmonary oedema.
    (b) cystic fibrosis.
    (c) pulmonary stenosis.
    (d) cigarette smoking.
    (e) bronchial obstruction.

118 Long-term effects of ionizing radiation include
    (a) telangiectasia.
    (b) vascular narrowing due to an endarteritis obliterans.
    (c) cystic medionecrosis.
    (d) skin atrophy.
    (e) squamous-cell carcinoma of the skin.

119 Metastatic calcification
    (a) develops in the presence of a normal calcium level in the blood.
    (b) often involves blood vessel walls.
    (c) usually indicates the presence of an epithelial neoplasm.
    (d) is usually detected by mammography.
    (e) is diagnostic of hyperparathyroidism.

120 In the amyloidoses
    (a) beta plicated sheets of modified starch molecules are laid down in connective tissue.
    (b) amyloid L only occurs in association with multiple myeloma.
    (c) rheumatoid arthritis predisposes to amyloid A.
    (d) the carpal tunnel syndrome is seen in beta-2-microglobulin-associated amyloid.
    (e) a diagnostic rectal biopsy needs to include submucosal vessels.

121 Factors which increase the risk of atheroma include:
    (a) the presence of a cholesteatoma.
    (b) high plasma levels of high-density lipoprotein.
    (c) systemic diastolic hypertension.
    (d) type B personality behaviour.
    (e) diabetes mellitus.

122 Superior mesenteric artery occlusion
    (a) is more common than normal in patients with atrial fibrillation.
    (b) often results in a pale infarct of the small intestine.
    (c) can occur without intestinal ischaemia.
    (d) is a recognized late complication of myocardial infarction.
    (e) usually results in intussusception.

117 (a) **True**   The accumulation of fluid in the alveoli predisposes to infection.
    (b) **True**   The abnormally viscid secretion predisposes to pneumonia.
    (c) **False**   Narrowing of the pulmonary valve does not make pneumonia more likely.
    (d) **True**   It interferes with alveolar macrophage function, causes chronic bronchitis and squamous metaplasia of the respiratory tract – all of which increase the likelihood of infection.
    (e) **True**   It tends to prevent the expulsion of potentially infective material from the lung.

118 (a) **True**   These may persist for many years.
    (b) **True**   Thought to be the result of damage to the intima.
    (c) **False**   This occurs in the aorta, for other reasons.
    (d) **True**   May be accompanied by depigmentation.
    (e) **True**   Other neoplasms are also more common.

119 (a) **False**   It is associated with hypercalcaemia.
    (b) **True**   This is one of the commoner sites where it is seen.
    (c) **False**   'Metastatic' does not refer to neoplasia in this term.
    (d) **False**   Dystrophic calcification (with a normal serum calcium) is often demonstrated by this technique.
    (e) **False**   It may be associated with any disease giving hypercalcaemia.

120 (a) **False**   The amyloids are protein molecules with a beta plicated sheet structure.
    (b) **False**   Light chain-associated amyloid is also seen with other forms of lymphoid neoplasia.
    (c) **True**   Amyloid A is derived from serum amyloid A, which is an acute phase protein abnormal in many inflammatory (and neoplastic) conditions.
    (d) **True**   This form of amyloid is seen in patients with chronic renal failure who are on dialysis.
    (e) **True**   A negative biopsy is inadequate if it does not include these.

121 (a) **False**   This condition of the ear is unrelated to atheroma.
    (b) **False**   HDL levels are inversely correlated. LDL levels are positively correlated.
    (c) **True**   This is a major risk factor.
    (d) **False**   There is some correlation with type A behaviour.
    (e) **True**   This is a major risk factor.

122 (a) **True**   Left atrial thrombus may embolize there.
    (b) **False**   Infarcts of the small intestine are congested red infarcts.
    (c) **True**   Slow occlusion, e.g. by atheroma, allows a collateral circulation to open up.
    (d) **True**   Mural thrombus from the left ventricle may embolize.
    (e) **False**   It is not an aetiological factor in intussusception.

123 Small pulmonary thrombo-emboli
   (a) do not cause pulmonary infarction in otherwise normal individuals.
   (b) may be organized by granulation tissue to fibrous tissue.
   (c) are a recognized cause of pulmonary hypertension.
   (d) most frequently originate in deep calf veins.
   (e) may be lysed by the pulmonary fibrinolytic system.

124 In a patient with a dissecting aneurysm
   (a) the lower abdominal aorta is the vessel most frequently affected.
   (b) the intima is dissected from the media by arterial blood.
   (c) haemopericardium is liable to occur.
   (d) infection is a common predisposing factor.
   (e) abnormal connective tissue is common in the aortic media.

125 In the blood vessels of patients with chronic type I diabetes mellitus
   (a) hyaline arteriolar sclerosis is usually a prominent feature.
   (b) arterio-venous aneurysms are frequently seen.
   (c) a granulomatous vasculitis is characteristically seen.
   (d) atheroma is often particularly severe.
   (e) there is increased glycosylation of basement membrane protein.

126 Concerning the cell cycle
   (a) the growth fraction in the tumour cell population is that proportion of the
       cells in the cell cycle.
   (b) the growth of tumours is usually associated with a marked shortening of cell
       cycle time.
   (c) in the G2 phase the cell has a diploid number of chromosomes.
   (d) growth of the cell is concentrated in the G1 and G2 phases.
   (e) in the S phase the amount of DNA in the cell is doubled.

127 Hyperplasia
   (a) only occurs in cell lines capable of mitosis.
   (b) is usually reversible.
   (c) usually indicates the presence of a neoplasm.
   (d) is an increase in the size of an organ or tissue due to an increase in cell
       size.
   (e) rarely occurs in patients over the age of 45 years.

128 A hamartoma
   (a) usually contains tissue from all three germ layers.
   (b) usually metastasizes via the blood stream.
   (c) is often present from birth.
   (d) may predispose to malignancy.
   (e) usually contains cells showing severe dysplasia.

123 (a) **True**   Usually cause true infarction only if the venous drainage of the lung is impaired.
    (b) **True**   They may leave residual fibrous tissue bands in the arteries.
    (c) **True**   Multiple small emboli may result in pulmonary hypertension.
    (d) **True**   Other sources include the pelvic veins.
    (e) **True**   They may leave no permanent lesion.

124 (a) **False**   The thoracic aorta is most frequently affected.
    (b) **False**   The dissection is in the media, separating it into inner and outer parts.
    (c) **True**   Cardiac tamponade may result from dissection back to the aortic root.
    (d) **False**   Infection is not usually involved in its development.
    (e) **True**   Abnormal amounts of glycosaminoglycans are present either in idiopathic cystic medionecrosis or in association with Marfan's syndrome.

125 (a) **True**   It is often severe.
    (b) **False**   Capillary microaneurysms may be present in the retina.
    (c) **False**   A granulomatous reaction is not a feature of vessels in diabetes mellitus.
    (d) **True**   And it often extends into smaller vessels than those where it is conventionally seen.
    (e) **True**   This contributes to basement membrane thickening and to diabetic microangiopathy.

126 (a) **True**   Estimates of this fraction may be obtained in different ways, such as measuring the labelling index.
    (b) **False**   This is usually near normal. Variation in cell birth rate or death rate may be more important.
    (c) **False**   Normal cells will have doubled their DNA content by the time G2 is reached.
    (d) **False**   'G' indicates 'gap' phases. G1 precedes the synthetic (S) phase and G2 precedes the mitotic (M) phase.
    (e) **True**   The activity of DNA polymerase results in doubling of the cell's DNA content.

127 (a) **True**   Permanent (or 'post-mitotic') cells cannot undergo hyperplasia.
    (b) **True**   Classically in hyperplasia, removal of the stimulus causing it results in reversion to normal. This is not always the case.
    (c) **False**   But persistent and severe hyperplasia may predispose to the development of a neoplasm.
    (d) **False**   This is hypertrophy.
    (e) **False**   Hyperplasia of some cell lines may occur at any age.

128 (a) **False**   A teratoma often shows this feature.
    (b) **False**   They are benign.
    (c) **True**   Though they may not present clinically until later in life.
    (d) **True**   Some may do, but usually they are quite benign.
    (e) **False**   The cells are usually normal.

129 In grading an adeno-carcinoma in the gastrointestinal tract the pathologist may take into consideration
    (a) pleomorphism of the cells.
    (b) the mitotic count.
    (c) invasion of the muscularis propria.
    (d) the presence of lymph node metastases.
    (e) the degree of gland formation.

130 Teratomas
    (a) may originate outside the gonads.
    (b) of the testis are unable to produce beta-HCG.
    (c) can be benign.
    (d) may show extra-embryonic differentiation.
    (e) have a peak incidence in the sixth decade.

131 In an undifferentiated malignant neoplasm found in an excised lymph node, immunohistochemistry for the following substances may help in identifying the tumour type
    (a) leucocyte common antigen (LCA).
    (b) laminin.
    (c) S100 protein.
    (d) prostatic acid phosphatase.
    (e) desmin.

132 The following lesions have a significantly increased risk of developing invasive carcinoma
    (a) Paget's disease of the nipple.
    (b) atrophic gastritis.
    (c) cirrhosis of the liver.
    (d) chronic peptic ulcer in the duodenum.
    (e) a tubular adenoma of the colon.

133 In carcinogenesis, oncogenes
    (a) are only involved in viral carcinogenesis.
    (b) are similar to normal growth control genes.
    (c) may be activated by translocation.
    (d) contribute to the malignant phenotype of neoplastic cells.
    (e) may code for growth factors or growth-factor receptors.

134 The following are well-documented associations of viruses and human malignancy:
    (a) human immunodeficiency virus (HIV) and B-cell lymphoma.
    (b) cytomegalovirus (CMV) and nasopharyngeal carcinoma.
    (c) Epstein-Barr virus (EBV) and Burkitt's lymphoma.
    (d) hepatitis A and hepatocellular carcinoma.
    (e) human papilloma virus (HPV) type 16 and squamous carcinoma of the cervix.

129 (a) **True** Variation in size and shape of the cells affects its degree of differentiation – which is grading.
(b) **True** This also affects grading.
(c) **False** This is a measurement of spread, which is staging, not grading.
(d) **False** This is also a factor affecting staging, not grading.
(e) **True** This gives a measure of differentiation in an adenocarcinoma.

130 (a) **True** Particularly in mid-line sites.
(b) **False** If there is trophoblastic differentiation, beta-HCG is produced.
(c) **True** The teratoma of the ovary (benign cystic teratoma or dermoid cyst) is characteristically benign.
(d) **True** Trophoblastic or yolk-sac differentiation may occur.
(e) **False** Commoner in earlier decades.

131 (a) **True** This is present in many lymphomas and not in epithelial tumours.
(b) **False** This is a basement membrane protein and its presence does not identify cell type.
(c) **True** This is present in many malignant melanomas. It can be present in other tumours and its significance has to be interpreted with other findings.
(d) **True** This is present in most adenocarcinomas of the prostate and has rarely been recorded elsewhere.
(e) **True** Is present in many smooth-muscle tumours.

132 (a) **True** There is usually an underlying ductal carcinoma, which is initially *in-situ* but then invasive.
(b) **True** Adenocarcinoma of the stomach tends to develop in an abnormal mucosa.
(c) **True** Especially with that due to hepatitis B but also with other forms. Hepatocellular carcinoma is more common.
(d) **False** Duodenal adenocarcinoma is very rare.
(e) **True** Both tubular and villous adenomas show dysplastic epithelium and are pre-malignant. The likelihood of invasive tumour being present at the time of removal increases with the size of the lesion.

133 (a) **False** They are involved in malignant neoplasms whatever the aetiology.
(b) **True** Proto-oncogenes (synonym: cellular oncogenes) are the equivalent in normal cells. If changed or abnormally activated they may become oncogenes.
(c) **True** Translocation of a proto-oncogene may result in its abnormal expression as an oncogene.
(d) **True** They are an essential part of the malignant phenotype.
(e) **True** They may also have other functions.

134 (a) **True** T-cell lymphoma and Hodgkin's disease have also been described in association with HIV but less frequently.
(b) **False** It is associated with EBV and 100% of these tumours contain EBV DNA.
(c) **True** About 98% of African Burkitt's contain EBV DNA but only about 20% of those originating outside Africa.
(d) **False** It is chronic hepatitis B virus (HBV) infection that is strongly associated.
(e) **True** This is the commonest type associated (about 50%) but others are also.

135 The following are known to predispose to the development of a cutaneous malignant melanoma
    (a) human papilloma virus infection.
    (b) xeroderma pigmentosum.
    (c) inherited defect of the retinoblastoma gene.
    (d) exposure to UV light.
    (e) melanosis coli.

136 Antibiotic prophylaxis of surgical wound infections
    (a) may usefully be started up to 6 hours after the operation.
    (b) should continue for at least 5 days after an operation.
    (c) reduces the infection rate for clean surgery to 5%.
    (d) is not indicated if the patient is already receiving antibiotics.
    (e) is unnecessary for procedures lasting less than 15 minutes.

137 *Clostridium difficile*-associated colitis is
    (a) diagnosed by culture of the organism from the stool.
    (b) characterized by the presence of the organism in blood culture.
    (c) frequently recurs after treatment.
    (d) associated with cross infection.
    (e) known to follow the use of amoxycillin.

138 Endotoxin is
    (a) the peptidoglycan component of bacterial cell walls.
    (b) produced by food-poisoning strains of *Staphylococcus aureus*.
    (c) an immunogen.
    (d) also known as tumour necrosis factor.
    (e) destroyed during steam sterilization of infusions.

135 (a) **False** There is no known association with malignant melanoma.
  (b) **True** This inherited defect of DNA repair mechanisms predisposes to skin neoplasia.
  (c) **False** This predisposes to the development of retinoblastoma.
  (d) **True** Excess exposure is associated with an increased risk of basal and squamous cell carcinoma as well as malignant melanoma.
  (e) **False** This disorder involves pigment deposition (not true melanin) in histiocytes in the colonic lamina propria and has nothing to do with melanoma.

136 (a) **False** Prophylaxis should begin before the operation, either with the premedication or ideally intravenously at induction of anaesthesia. The use of antibiotics after the operation is early treatment of infection rather than prophylaxis or prevention.
  (b) **False** One to three doses is sufficient.
  (c) **False** The infection rate for clean surgery should be less than 5% irrespective of antimicrobial prophylaxis.
  (d) **False** Infection may occur with organisms resistant to current therapy.
  (e) **False** For example, instrumentation of sites either infected or heavily colonized with bacteria can produce a septicaemia, which may be prevented by antibiotic prophylaxis.

137 (a) **False** *Clostridium difficile* may be isolated from healthy carriers. The diagnosis requires the detection of *C.difficile* cytotoxin.
  (b) **False** *Clostridium difficile* is very rarely invasive.
  (c) **True** Relapses are common (10–20%) and may require repeated courses of therapy.
  (d) **True** Particularly in institutions for the elderly.
  (e) **True** Although originally associated mainly with the use of clindamycin, most antibiotics have been associated with this condition.

138 (a) **False** It is the lipopolysaccharide component of Gram-negative bacterial cell membranes.
  (b) **False** Food-poisoning strains of *Staphylococcus aureus* produce and export from the cell a protein enterotoxin.
  (c) **True** Endotoxin evokes an immune response. Monoclonal antibody directed against the core region of endotoxin appears to reduce mortality in endotoxic shock.
  (d) **False** Tumour necrosis factor (also known as cachectin) is a cytokine produced by a variety of human cells and is an important mediator of septic shock.
  (e) **False** Endotoxin is heat-stable and endotoxic shock may follow infusion of solutions contaminated with Gram-negative bacteria even if the fluid has been sterilized and the bacteria are no longer viable.

139 Infection with hepatitis B virus
   (a) usually has an incubation period of 2–3 weeks.
   (b) is required for hepatitis C infection.
   (c) may be transmitted from surgeon to patient during surgery.
   (d) is unlikely to be transmissible once a patient has antibodies to surface antigen.
   (e) is prevented by a live attenuated vaccine.

140 Beta-haemolytic streptococci group A (*Strep. pyogenes*)
   (a) produce a characteristic beta-lactamase.
   (b) are one of the causes of necrotizing fasciitis.
   (c) are the most common cause of infective endocarditis.
   (d) are part of the normal vaginal flora.
   (e) may be carried asymptomatically in the throat.

141 Coagulase-negative staphylococci
   (a) cause community-acquired urinary tract infection.
   (b) are the commonest cause of wound infection after clean surgery.
   (c) may readily be distinguished from Staphylococcus aureus on the basis of a Gram stain.
   (d) adhere to plastic materials by production of extracellular slime.
   (e) are part of the normal flora of the axilla.

142 Patients who carry multiple (methicillin-)resistant *Staphylococcus aureus* (MRSA)
   (a) should not undergo surgery until the organism has been eradicated.
   (b) often harbour the organism in the nose.
   (c) must be nursed in barrier isolation.
   (d) should be treated with intravenous mupirocin.
   (e) may be managed safely in the community.

139 (a) **False** The average incubation period is from 60–90 days, but ranges from 45–180 days.

    (b) **False** Coexistent hepatitis B infection is required for hepatitis D (delta agent) infection, a defective RNA-containing virus. Hepatitis C is usually transmitted by blood transfusion.

    (c) **True** This has occurred with dentists, oral surgeons and obstetricians and gynaecologists who are hepatitis B virus carriers.

    (d) **True** Antibody to hepatitis B surface antigen is a reliable indicator of non-infectivity.

    (e) **False** The most commonly used hepatitis B vaccine consists of surface antigen manufactured by recombinant DNA techniques and is not a live vaccine.

140 (a) **False** *Strep. pyogenes* does not produce any beta-lactamase (penicillinase).

    (b) **True** These organisms may produce a gangrenous cellulitis with bullae and penetration of fascial planes.

    (c) **False** The viridans streptococci are the common cause of infective endocarditis.

    (d) **False** Lancefield group B streptococci (also known as *Streptococcus agalactiae*) are part of the normal vaginal flora.

    (e) **True** The organism may also be carried in the nose and on skin. Outbreaks of *Strep. pyogenes* infection in surgical patients have been traced to operating theatre staff carrying the organism.

141 (a) **True** The most common example being *Staphylococcus saprophyticus* which characteristically causes acute urinary tract infection in young women.

    (b) **False** *Staph. aureus* (coagulase positive) is the commonest cause of wound infection after clean surgery.

    (c) **False** They are indistinguishable on the basis of a Gram stain. The coagulase test distinguishes these two groups.

    (d) **True** Particularly intravascular catheters, vascular and other prostheses.

    (e) **True** And most of the rest of the integument.

142 (a) **False** The presence of the organism should not rule out essential surgery although for some elective procedures it may be desirable to eradicate carriage.

    (b) **True** This is a useful site to sample when screening for carriage.

    (c) **False** This is not essential, particularly for trivial infection or a low degree of colonization.

    (d) **False** Mupirocin is available for topical use only.

    (e) **True** They represent no serious hazard.

143 Active immunization is advised
   (a) against tetanus in a patient who has recovered from the disease.
   (b) following splenectomy for trauma in an otherwise healthy individual.
   (c) for hospital staff who perform mouth to mouth resuscitation of a patient with meningococcal meningitis.
   (d) against *Clostridium perfringens* for a surgeon after a needle-stick injury during surgery for gas gangrene.
   (e) for a surgeon who has incised a neck abscess subsequently shown to be tuberculous.

144 Bacterial causes of diarrhoea
   (a) acquired in hospital include *Clostridium botulinum*.
   (b) may be associated with arthropathy.
   (c) can usefully be diagnosed by electron microscopy.
   (d) should not be treated with antibiotics.
   (e) include several zoonoses.

145 Disinfectants
   (a) possess little selective toxicity.
   (b) become progressively more active at higher concentrations.
   (c) cause hypersensitivity reactions.
   (d) are inactivated by organic material.
   (e) are more active when used in combination.

143 (a) **True**   Tetanus does not result in natural immunity to reinfection.
    (b) **True**   Such patients are otherwise at risk of overwhelming capsulated bacterial infection, such as pneumococci and should receive pneumococcal vaccine.
    (c) **False**   Antibiotic prophylaxis (with ciprofloxacin or rifampicin) is advised.
    (d) **False**   This is not necessary and there is no vaccine against this organism. There may, of course, be a risk of hepatitis B.
    (e) **False**   The risk of transmission is negligible.

144 (a) **False**   *Clostridium perfringens* may cause diarrhoea (and vomiting).
    (b) **True**   Reactive arthropathy is particularly associated with Yersinia enterocolitica, but may also follow infection with *Salmonella spp.*
    (c) **False**   This is suitable only for the diagnosis of viral causes, such as rotavirus.
    (d) **False**   For example *Salmonella spp.* (food-poisoning types) and Shigella species infections may be treated with the new 4-quinolone antibiotics.
    (e) **True**   Campylobacter and the food-poisoning types of salmonella are usually derived ultimately from animal sources.

145 (a) **True**   They are usually active against a range of microorganisms.
    (b) **False**   At high concentrations activity declines.
    (c) **True**   Particularly the aldehyde compounds such as glutaraldehyde.
    (d) **True**   Hence the need for thorough cleaning of instruments before disinfection.
    (e) **False**   In many instances combinations result in loss of activity.

4 Surgery in General

146 Burns
   (a) from an electrical injury are not serious if the skin wound is slight.
   (b) in house fires fluid depletion is the cause of loss of consciousness.
   (c) in a limb, always require escharotomies.
   (d) with smoke inhalation require immediate tracheostomy.
   (e) around the face are best managed by an occlusive dressing.

147 In a patient presenting with a head injury
   (a) a dilated pupil immediately after the injury is a relevant neurological sign.
   (b) who smells of alcohol, a skull radiograph should be performed.
   (c) a CT scan is routinely performed.
   (d) requiring an emergency standard temporal burr hole, the dura should be opened if an extradural clot is not present.
   (e) and CSF rhinorrhoea should be treated with prophylactic antibiotics.

148 In a patient with a diffuse unilateral swelling of the parotid gland
   (a) a pleomorphic adenoma is the most likely cause.
   (b) pain and tenderness at mastication discriminate between a benign and a malignant lesion.
   (c) sialography should be considered.
   (d) a fine needle aspirate is crucial for the diagnosis.
   (e) computerized tomography is routinely performed.

146 (a) **False**   Damage to the deeper tissues, blood vessels, muscles and the myocardium may later become apparent.

   (b) **False**   Unconsciousness is caused by inhalation of poisonous gases such as the gas produced from burning polyurethane foam products (isocyanates), ammonia, nitric oxide or carbon monoxide.

   (c) **False**   Escharotomies are required only if a full thickness burn encircles the limb because of the risk of ischaemic contracture or gangrene.

   (d) **False**   The treatment for suspected respiratory tract burns include oxygen mask, physiotherapy, bronchodilators, steroids and endotracheal intubation. Tracheostomy should only be carried out if intubation is difficult or prolonged.

   (e) **False**   These are best left open to avoid eye damage by medication and crusting of the dressings.

147 (a) **False**   This is usually due to traumatic mydriasis when neither pupil can then be used as a guide to lateralization.

   (b) **True**   It is difficult to assess patients when under the effect of alcohol. Other indications for radiography include loss of consciousness and amnesia, neurological symptoms or signs, penetrating injury and scalp bruising or swelling.

   (c) **False**   The indications for CT scanning are: persistent headache, deterioration in level of consciousness, confusion or neurological deficit with or without skull fractures.

   (d) **False**   This is unwise and it is more reasonable to make a frontal or parietal hole.

   (e) **True**   Antibiotics are initially required to avoid the risk of meningitis. Several factors are taken into consideration before advising surgery.

148 (a) **False**   A pleomorphic ademona is a discrete lump in the region of the parotid gland. Diffuse swelling can be due to sialadenitis secondary to obstruction, viral and bacterial infection, or auto-immune disease.

   (b) **True**   Viral and bacterial parotiditis and sialolithiasis, cause recurrent fever, pain and tenderness particularly at mastication that are not present with malignant lesions.

   (c) **True**   A calculus in the parotid duct would cause obstruction, which may be identified, and features of sialadenitis will show on the sialogram – both conditions cause diffuse swelling of the glands.

   (d) **False**   When a swelling is discrete, superficial parotidectomy without pre-operative biopsy is the appropriate approach as pleomorphic adenoma is the most likely cause. With a diffuse swelling where sialography has failed to identify the cause, an open biopsy is preferable. Needle biopsy may result in tumour seedling, misdiagnosis because of sampling error and injury to surrounding structures.

   (e) **False**   CT scanning is necessary only if there are signs that the swelling is infiltrating the deeper structures or bone. It would outline the extent of the disease for planning treatment.

149 A multinodular goitre
   (a) is common in puberty.
   (b) with secondary hyperthyroidism causes ophthalmic signs.
   (c) should be suspected to be malignant if it is rapidly enlarging.
   (d) requiring surgery preoperatively laryngoscopy is unnecessary unless there
       is hoarseness of voice.
   (e) is better treated by total rather than subtotal thyroidectomy.

150 In a blunt injury to the chest
   (a) pulsus paradoxus is an alarming sign.
   (b) comparing the blood pressure in the upper limbs is of no relevance.
   (c) subcutaneous emphysema is only seen if the injury is penetrating.
   (d) with a flail chest, this should be treated by skeletal fixation.
   (e) the presence of a haemothorax demands immediate thoracotomy.

151 In mammary dysplasia
   (a) a discrete lump is commonly a fibroadenoma.
   (b) breast lumpiness is bilateral.
   (c) a spiculated irregular margin on a mammogram should arouse suspicion.
   (d) symptomatic treatment of a painful lump is excision.
   (e) screening is necessary because of cancer risk.

149 (a) **False** At puberty an increased demand for thyroid hormones causes diffuse swelling of the gland.

(b) **False** These signs are the hallmarks of Graves' Disease, which is the classic thyrotoxicosis associated with a diffuse not a nodular goitre.

(c) **True** Malignant change occurs in 5% of untreated multinodular goiters. Other suspicious features are adjacent lymph node enlargement or a recurrent laryngeal nerve palsy.

(d) **False** 3–5% patients are found to have paresis or paralysis of the vocal cords due to neuritis following exanthemata during childhood, which is worth documenting before thyroidectomy for medico-legal reasons.

(e) **False** The morbidity with subtotal thyroidectomy is less, and even if a few nodules remain in the remnant, recurrent goitre is rare.

150 (a) **True** This indicates cardiac tamponade as a result of pericardial or myocardial damage causing bleeding into the pericardial cavity.

(b) **False** Traumatic rupture of the aorta may complicate such an injury and usually takes place at or near the origin of the left subclavian artery, so the blood pressure in the left arm is appreciably lower than in the right.

(c) **False** Laceration of the lung by a fractured rib causes emphysema over the site of injury or air may pass beneath the visceral pleura, via the mediastinum and appear in the neck.

(d) **False** Except for minor degrees of unstable chest wall, positive-pressure ventilation through an endotracheal tube or a trache-ostomy may be required and has superceded sugical treatment.

(e) **False** Should initially be drained with an intercostal chest drain but if the bleeding continues thoracotomy is indicated.

151 (a) **True** Diffuse lumpiness also occurs in mammary dysplasia.

(b) **True** The lumpiness may be symmetrical in the upper outer quadrants of both sides, and less commonly confined to one quadrant of one breast.

(c) **True** Microcalcifications, branching or in irregular form, arranged in cluster or ductal distribution on a mamogram are other suspi-cious features.

(d) **False** Reassurance, analgesia, primrose-oil, prolactin inhibitors, e.g. bromocriptine or danazol, and anti-oestrogens, e.g. tamoxifen, are the treatment options.

(e) **False** Mammary dysplasia is not particularly a premalignant condition. Regular mammography will be determined by the clinical course. Screening, like in other women, would be unnecessary before the age of 50 years.

152 Reflux oesophagitis
  (a) is always associated with a hiatus hernia.
  (b) causes melaena stool.
  (c) producing an oesophageal stricture is an indication for surgery.
  (d) predisposes to squamous cell carcinoma of the oesophagus.
  (e) is best treated by an anti-reflux procedure.

153 Duodenal ulceration
  (a) is cured by H2 antagonists.
  (b) endoscopy and multiple biopsies before and after treatment are required.
  (c) can be determined to be due to hypergastrinaemia by measuring the maximum acid output to pentagastrin stimulation.
  (d) partial gastrectomy is the first line of treatment for acute bleeding.
  (e) highly selective vagotomy is the preferred type of vagotomy because of its low recurrence rate.

154 In a patient presenting with jaundice
  (a) an ultrasound examination is an essential early investigation.
  (b) an ERCP should always be performed.
  (c) complicated with cholangitis surgical intervention is urgently demanded.
  (d) when due to bile duct stones sphincterotomy without cholecystectomy is adequate treatment in the elderly patient.
  (e) and requiring surgery, diuretics should be given preoperatively in order to prevent renal failure.

152 (a) **False** While most patients (80%) with clinically significant reflux have a hiatus hernia, reflux can occur in the absence of a hernia. At least half the patients with hiatus hernia are asymptomatic.

(b) **True** Can cause acute or chronic bleeding with iron deficiency anaemia.

(c) **False** Endoscopic dilatation combined with H2 antagonists or a proton pump inhibitor is often adequate treatment.

(d) **False** Reflux oesophagitis may progress to a Barrett's oesophagus (migration of glandular epithelium at the cardio-oesophageal junction) proximally, which may progress to adenocarcinoma.

(e) **False** Reducing weight, avoiding smoking, light garments, raising the head of the bed and using H2 and proton pump-inhibitors are quite effective in controlling patients' symptoms.

153 (a) **False** Medical treatment controls symptoms and heals ulceration but does not cure an ulcer; relapses frequently occur on cessation of treatment.

(b) **False** Initial diagnostic endoscopy is sufficient. The symptomatic response is an adequate measure of healing. As there is no risk of malignancy (unlike gastric ulcers) tissue diagnosis is not essential.

(c) **False** Fasting serum gastrin is the diagnostic measurement.

(d) **False** Surgery should only be considered if initial treatment by endoscopic sclerotherapy, or heat or laser coagulation has failed. Besides, a vagotomy with under-running of the bleeding vessel is the preferable procedure because of its lower immediate and long-term morbidity.

(e) **False** It is preferred because of the low risk of dumping and diarrhoea, but the recurrence rate as with truncal vagotomy is operator-dependent and can be similar.

154 (a) **True** The management is dependent on whether the cause of jaundice is intra- or extra-hepatic and this is determined by the absence or presence of extra-hepatic dilated bile ducts. Ultrasound examination will also show the level and perhaps the cause of obstruction.

(b) **False** ERCP is reserved to patients with an obstructed biliary tree demonstrated by ultrasound examination.

(c) **False** Blood culture and antibiotics could control the infection. Endoscopic or percutaneous drainage may be advisable should the infection fail to resolve. Surgery is the last resort.

(d) **True** Cholecystectomy can be deferred unless the patient's symptoms persist.

(e) **False** A forced diuresis will not protect the kidney from a possible hepatorenal syndrome (kidney failure in jaundiced patients). What is needed is adequate hydration by instituting intravenous fluids during and after the period of starvation.

155 In acute pancreatitis
  (a) minimal degree of hypoxia is common.
  (b) an ultrasound examination is routinely required.
  (c) due to gallstones, endoscopic sphincterotomy is recommended.
  (d) when complicated by a pseudocyst, early internal drainage is required.
  (e) serum calcium levels can be high.

156 In pancreatic carcinoma
  (a) patients commonly present with an abdominal mass.
  (b) patients infrequently suffer from gastric outlet obstruction.
  (c) angiography is essential for staging.
  (d) initial biliary drainage reduces the morbidity of a subsequent definitive procedure.
  (e) palliative surgical bypass is the optimal therapeutic option for advanced disease.

157 In acute small-bowel obstruction
  (a) early constipation is followed by distension, abdominal pain and vomiting.
  (b) examination of the abdominal wall for incision scars is necessary.
  (c) a barium follow-through would confirm the diagnosis.
  (d) localized guarding on abdominal examination would require urgent laparotomy.
  (e) due to adhesions, division would obviate the risk of further obstruction.

158 In acute left-sided colonic obstruction
  (a) sigmoid volvulus is the commonest cause.
  (b) sigmoidoscopy is necessary if volvulus is suspected.
  (c) distension and tenderness in the right iliac fossa are ominous signs.
  (d) an instant contrast enema is an essential part of the management.
  (e) a defunctioning colostomy is the standard treatment.

155 (a) **True** This is due to several factors, retroperitoneal oedema, elevation of the diaphragm, reduced ventilation because of pain, pleural effusion, right to left shunting of blood, intravascular coagulation in the lungs, loss of pulmonary surfactant and increased affinity of oxyhaemoglobin for oxygen.

(b) **True** This is to confirm pancreatic oedema and demonstrate whether calculi in the gall bladder or bile ducts are present.

(c) **True** This has proven to be a safe and effective treatment for decompressing the biliary tree.

(d) **False** About half of all the cases are complicated by the formation of pseudocysts and 20–40% of these resolve spontaneously. Therefore, any intervention should not be considered before a few months of observation unless the cyst is causing symptoms.

(e) **True** Although with a severe attack the serum calcium falls, hypercalcaemia can be the cause of acute pancreatitis and should, therefore, be investigated.

156 (a) **False** The commonest site of a carcinoma is the head of the pancreas. Jaundice due to biliary obstruction precedes the appearance of a mass in most cases.

(b) **True** The pyloroduodenal region is obstructed by tumour in 15% of patients with carcinoma in the head of the pancreas.

(c) **False** CT scanning provides adequate visualization of the tumour boundaries, the venous outline and lymph-node enlargement.

(d) **False** Biliary drainage has its complications without an appreciable improvement in morbidity following major definitive surgery.

(e) **False** Unless there is an associated gastric-outlet obstruction, endoscopic prosthesis is preferable.

157 (a) **False** With small bowel obstruction, vomiting and abdominal colic are earlier signs followed by distension and constipation.

(b) **True** Adhesions from previous surgery are the commonest cause of small bowel obstruction.

(c) **False** A plain abdominal x-ray is diagnostic if it shows dilated loops of small bowel. The level is determined by the number and pattern of fluid levels. A barium meal is contra-indicated.

(d) **True** This is a sign of internal strangulation and may proceed to intestinal infarction.

(e) **False** The risk increases. Conservative treatment by gastrointestinal decompression with a nasogastric tube is often successful and avoids surgery.

158 (a) **False** Diverticular disease and carcinoma are the usual causes of colonic obstruction.

(b) **True** This successfully decompresses the sigmoid and relieves obstruction avoiding the need for laparotomy.

(c) **True** With compentent ileo-caecal valve, distension of the caecum with perforation may result.

(d) **True** In order to exclude pseudo-obstruction especially in medically unfit patients, and to determine the site of obstruction.

(e) **False** Left-sided resection with or without primary anastomosis is increasingly being performed in order to avoid multi-staged procedures. A transverse colostomy is acceptable if the surgeon is inexperienced or the patient unfit.

159 In the case of an elderly lady presenting with a painful firm mass in the right lower abdomen and a temperature
   (a) an appendicular inflammatory mass is the only possible diagnosis.
   (b) antimicrobial therapy should be instituted.
   (c) an instant barium enema would establish the diagnosis.
   (d) colonoscopy after complete recovery is often advisable.
   (e) laparotomy would be necessary should the mass fail to resolve.

160 In diverticular disease
   (a) the whole colon is commonly involved.
   (b) a barium enema reliably identifies a carcinoma in a diseased segment.
   (c) a paracolic abscess often drains into the vagina.
   (d) cystoscopy is the investigation of choice in the diagnosis of a colo-vesical fistula.
   (e) surgery is recommended after an episode of acute diverticulitis.

161 An adult patient presenting with persistent severe rectal bleeding
   (a) should first have an upper gastrointestinal endoscopy.
   (b) requires an emergency barium enema examination.
   (c) should undergo colonoscopy if a barium enema fails to establish the diagnosis.
   (d) requires angiography if the source of bleeding is not identified.
   (e) would require total colectomy if sigmoid diverticula are found at an emergency laparotomy.

159 (a) **False** Caecal carcinoma, paracaecal inflammation secondary to tumour perforation, or associated appendicitis, sigmoid or caecal diverticulitis and rarely Crohn's disease can have a similar presentation.

(b) **True** The management of an inflammatory mass is by administration of antimicrobials and intravenous fluids with observation of vital signs.

(c) **False** With an inflammatory process associated with the large bowel, a barium enema should be avoided as it may cause a perforation. It is of no diagnostic value as any distortion in the outline of the caecum or the ascending colon could be related to extrinsic compression by the inflammatory reaction.

(d) **True** A barium enema may still fail to outline the caecum adequately for the reasons already mentioned. Colonoscopy allows better visualization of the caecum as it is necessary to exclude a carcinoma in this age group.

(e) **True** An inflammatory mass, particularly if related to acute appendicitis, usually resolves on antibiotic treatment. Exploration is necessary should the mass persist.

160 (a) **False** In nearly 60% of patients the disease is confined to the sigmoid colon. Total involvement occurs only in 10%.

(b) **False** A polyp or a carcinoma in a segment of diverticular disease is not always clearly outlined on a barium enema. Besides, the narrowing due to either can be difficult to differentiate. Endoscopy is, therefore, frequently necessary.

(c) **True** Unless drained surgically, the abscess drains into the vagina forming a colo-vaginal fistula.

(d) **True** An intravenous urogram or a barium enema does not reliably identify the fistula.

(e) **False** The risk of further complications is small to justify prophylatic surgery.

161 (a) **False** It is unlikely for a patient with a lesion in the upper gastrointestinal tract to present with massive rectal bleeding without haematemesis.

(b) **False** In an unprepared bowel, faecal residue would not permit adequate visualization of the colon. A barium enema is an unsuitable investigation for visualizing mucosal vascular malformations and the presence of barium would interfere with further imaging should the patient require angiography.

(c) **False** It is practically not possible to prepare the bowel for colonoscopy. Faecal residue and blood in the colon would also not allow clear visualization of the colon.

(d) **True** In a patient who continues to bleed, and in the light of difficulties in achieving a satisfactory diagnostic result with either barium enema or colonoscopy, angiography should be the standard investigation. Angiography will confirm the site of haemorrhage in at least 25% of patients, particularly with angiodysplasia, which is common in the elderly patient.

(e) **True** Left colonic resection might fail to control the bleeding unless this site has been determined by angiography as the sole source of bleeding, otherwise angiodysplasia in the right colon might be missed. This accounts for the high re-bleeding rate after left hemicolectomy performed for presumably bleeding sigmoid diverticular disease.

162 Colonic polyps
(a) are all premalignant.
(b) risk of malignancy is determined by both the size and the histological features in adenomatous polyps.
(c) when pedunculated are treated by colotomy and polypectomy.
(d) present in numbers of 10–20 are diagnostic of familial adenomatous polyposis.
(e) Occuring as familial adenomatous polyposis require proctocolectomy.

163 With a rectal carcinoma at 7 cms
(a) diagnosed by sigmoidoscopy and biopsy, a barium enema is unnecessary.
(b) the presence of liver secondaries would not preclude surgical resection.
(c) survival is better following abdomino-perineal excision than anterior resection.
(d) impotence can be a complication of rectal resection.
(e) postoperative radiotherapy is of no value.

164 Splenectomy
(a) is routinely performed in staging non-Hodgkin's lymphoma.
(b) for hereditary spherocytosis is sometimes combined with cholecystectomy.
(c) is an effective cure for idiopathic thrombocytopenic purpura.
(d) is commonly complicated by left basal atelectasis.
(e) should be preceded by pneumococcal antitoxin immunization.

165 An intra-abdominal abscess following laparotomy
(a) is more common if the surgical procedure involves a splenectomy.
(b) is a cause of paralytic ileus.
(c) is easily diagnosed by a plain abdominal x-ray.
(d) causes hypoproteinaemia.
(e) is only effectively treated by open drainage.

162 (a) **False**   Only adenomatous polyps may develop into carcinoma.
    (b) **True**   For adenomatous polyps larger than 1 cm the risk is about 10% and this reaches 50% in polyps more than 2 cm and histologically villous.
    (c) **False**   Endoscopic polypectomy is the conventional approach unless for technical reasons the polyp can not be safely snared.
    (d) **False**   The diagnosis is confidently made if there are more than 100 polyps that are histologically adenomas.
    (e) **False**   Total colectomy and ileorectal anastomosis with regular examination of the rectal pump and snaring of residual polyps avoids a permanent ileostomy. Patients unlikely to attend for this treatment, restorative proctocolectomy with ileoanal anastomosis should be considered.

163 (a) **False**   The colon should be fully visualized to exclude synchronous polyps or carcinoma, which may occur in 5% of patients.
    (b) **True**   Palliative resection should still be carried out for symptomatic relief and in order to avoid the risk of bleeding or obstruction.
    (c) **False**   The outcome after either treatment is comparable. Anterior resection avoids a colostomy.
    (d) **True**   Damage to the pelvic nerves during dissection may also result in bladder dysfunction.
    (e) **False**   Adjuvant radiotherapy or combined therapy with chemotherapy would reduce the risk of local recurrence and improve survival particularly in Dukes C disease.

164 (a) **False**   The accuracy of imaging in staging has superceded open laparotomy and splenectomy adds no advantage to the treatment.
    (b) **True**   Nearly 70% of untreated patients over the age of 10 years have pigment gallstones. Every child with gallstones should be investigated for evidence of hereditary spherocytosis.
    (c) **False**   60% can be regarded as cured, 20% will be improved and 15% will find no benefit from splenectomy.
    (d) **True**   This is due to damage or irritation of the left hemidiaphragm or a subphrenic abscess.
    (e) **True**   Splenectomized patients are at risk of septicaemia due to *Streptococcus pneumoniae*, *Neisseria meningitides* and *Haemophilus influenzae*. There is a better response to active immunization before the spleen is removed. Long-term antibiotic prophylaxis with penicillin is also necessary.

165 (a) **True**   Splenectomy is associated with a high morbidity due to sepsis particularly in cancer surgery.
    (b) **True**   Paralytic ileus in the presence of a temperature, a raised white cell count and normal electrolytes, intra-abdominal sepsis should be considered.
    (c) **False**   An abscess collection is demonstrated on a plain film only if gas-forming organisms produce a fluid level, although air in the early postoperative period may show similar features. Ultrasound and definitely CT scanning are better diagnostic methods.
    (d) **True**   Protein exudate and excessive catabolism associated with sepsis leads to a negative nitrogen balance.
    (e) **False**   Percutaenous drainage under radiological screening avoids re-exploration and wherever feasible is a better option.

166 In an inguinal hernia
  (a) herniorrhaphy is essential in a child.
  (b) irreducibility is a sign of strangulation.
  (c) differentiation between a direct and an indirect hernia is irrelevant in the patient's management.
  (d) excision of the sac is always performed.
  (e) scrotal haematoma is a complication of surgical repair.

167 In ureteric colic caused by a stone
  (a) diagnosis is confidently made by a plain x-ray film.
  (b) idiopathic hypercalcaemia is the commonest underlying metabolic disorder.
  (c) conservative treatment is adopted even if there is no progress of the stone down the ureter.
  (d) in the upper third of the ureter the choice of treatment is ureterolithotomy.
  (e) in the lower third and 1 cm in size it is removed by the Dormia basket.

168 Bladder carcinoma
  (a) should be considered as a possible diagnosis in a patient with prostatism.
  (b) is best staged by an open biopsy.
  (c) is often multiple and superficial, therefore, adjuvant radiotherapy is combined with endoscopic resection.
  (d) with muscle invasion is treated by preoperative radiotherapy and cystectomy.
  (e) ureterosigmoidostomy after cystectomy predisposes to colonic tumours.

166 (a) **False** This is a congenital hernia due to a patent processus vaginalis, therefore, a herniotomy is sufficient.

(b) **False** Extraperitoneal fat or omentum in the hernial sac may be entrapped within the inguinal canal rendering the hernia irreducible without necessarily involving the small bowel.

(c) **False** It is always necessary to be able to differentiate between a direct and an indirect hernia because the high risk of strangulation in an indirect inguinal hernia is sufficient reason for urging operation.

(d) **False** The sac in a direct hernia is small, the hernial mass consists of extraperitoneal fat, therefore, the sac is not removed. It is easily inverted into the abdomen and the transversalis fascia repaired in front of it.

(e) **True** Control of the superficial pudental and superficial epigastric vessels and adequate haemostasis in inguinoscrotal hernias, where the hernial sac is densely adherent to scrotal tissues, are necessary in avoiding this complication.

167 (a) **False** A small stone may not clearly show, while an opacity on a plain film is not necessarily a stone. An emergency intravenous urogram is required.

(b) **False** Idiopathic hypercalcurea rather than hypercalcaemia is a more common disorder, hence 24 hour urine for calcium and phosphate as well as serum calcium measurements should be performed.

(c) **False** Other indications for active intervention are persistent pain, evidence of renal functional impairment, or if there is infection above the site of obstruction.

(d) **False** Percutaneous removal and extracorporeal shock wave would avoid surgery and are currently more popular techniques

(e) **False** This is a hazardous technique that may damage the ureter when dealing with stones larger than 0.5 cm. Shattering the stone with a pulse dye laser or ultrasound is a better alternative treatment.

168 (a) **True** Infiltration of the bladder neck and prostate will cause symptoms of bladder outlet obstruction.

(b) **False** There is no place for open biopsy because of the danger of wound implantation. Biopsy with cystoscopic forceps is inadequate for staging as only the superficial part of the tumour is sampled. Transurethral resection and examination under anaesthesia allow adequate clinical staging.

(c) **False** For superficial tumours radiotherapy is ineffective: topical chemotherapy can be used to treat residual multifocal deposits. Occasionally cystectomy is the only possible treatment when multifocal superficial disease cannot be controlled by local resection and chemotherapy.

(d) **True** Nodal metastasis occurs in 40% of patients with invasive disease which is reduced to 20% when preoperative radiotherapy is administered. Radical external beam radiotherapy with salvage cystectomy when tumour persists or recurs is an acceptable alternative option.

(e) **True** For this reason patients should have regular colonoscopy. Ureterosigmoidostomy also causes ascending infection, reabsorption of urea and chloride, chronic metabolic acidosis and incontinence of fluid faeces.

169 In the case of a young adult with a firm and enlarged testicle
   (a) the patient should be warned that this could only be a testicular tumour.
   (b) a testicular tumour is confirmed by orchidectomy through a scrotal incision.
   (c) high serum α-fetoprotein and β-human chorionic gonadotrophin is of clinical value.
   (d) which proves to be a Stage I seminoma, adjuvant retroperitoneal node irradiation is the usual practice.
   (e) which proves to be a Stage I teratoma, orchidectomy and retroperitoneal wide dissection offers the best therapeutic result.

170 With a urethral disruption after a pelvic injury
   (a) the pelvic ring is commonly fractured.
   (b) difficulty in palpating the prostate suggests that the bladder and prostate have been displaced.
   (c) percutaneous suprapubic catheterization is safer than urethral catheterization.
   (d) the railroad technique has no place in the treatment.
   (e) failure of erection is the ultimate outcome in half the patients.

171 In an abdominal aortic aneurysm
   (a) the femoral pulses are often equal and palpable even with ruptured aneurysm.
   (b) an aortogram is essential to establish the diagnosis.
   (c) elective surgery is indicated if on clinical examination the vessel diameter is more than 7 cms.
   (d) unclamping the aorta after the repair can cause cardiac arrhythmia.
   (e) following repair, haematemesis is a recognized presentation.

169 (a) **False** Differential diagnosis includes epididymitis, torsion of the testis, tuberculosis, gumma and granulomatous orchitis.

(b) **False** An inguinal approach allows ligating the testicular blood vessels before handling the tumour. Incising the scrotum breaches the tunica albugina and predisposes to local recurrence and opens another pathway of lymphatic spread.

(c) **True** This is diagnostic of a testicular tumour, of its extent and response to treatment.

(d) **True** The exquisite radiosensitivity of the tumour and the rarity of wide metastatic spread have made this approach logical.

(e) **False** Orchidectomy with or without retroperitoneal node treatment by excision or radiotherapy are equally successful. The risk of ejaculatory impotence after retroperitoneal node dissection has made this approach unpopular. Surveillance following orchidectomy reduces morbidity; though there is recurrence of 25%, the surveillance policy detects this while the metastases are of small volume and curable.

170 (a) **True** When the pubic bones and their rami or the centre of the pelvic ring or the innominate bone on one side of the pelvic ring is displaced backwards, the prostate is pulled from the ischial rami, to which are attached the corpora cavernosa and thereby the bulbar urethra, shearing the membranous urethra.

(b) **False** A large haematoma around the prostate may make it impalpable.

(c) **True** Urethral catheterization carries the risk of converting an incomplete rupture of the urethra, which may well heal without a stricture, into a complete rupture that will inevitably heal with stricture formation.

(d) **False** When the rupture is complete, railroading a catheter across the gap and drawing the prostate down to the triangular ligament is adopted particularly if a laparotomy is undertaken because of other injuries.

(e) **True** Whether this is due to damage to the pelvic parasympathetic nerves, damage to the arterial supply to the erectile tissue or damage to both is not clear.

171 (a) **True** In cases of rupture, the pulse may be suppressed by the surrounding haematoma, but in dissecting aneurysms, side branch ostia are sheared and closed, resulting in absence of distal pulses.

(b) **False** A plain radiograph may show a line of calcification in the aneurysmal wall and an ultrasound examination is diagnostic. An aortogram is only indicated if it is suspected clinically that the renal arteris are involved.

(c) **True** A 5 cm diameter aneurysm is a critical threshold. The risk of rupture is 25% when the diameter is less than 7 cm and 46% in those which are 7–10 cm in diameter. Larger aneurysms have a 60% risk of rupture.

(d) **True** Clamping the aorta causes tissue ischaemia and metabolic acidosis. The metabolites are flushed into the circulation when the aorta is unclamped.

(e) **True** An aortic prosthetic graft may erode into the duodenum creating an aorto-duodenal fistula.

172 In acute ischaemia of the leg
   (a) early loss of function suggests an embolus.
   (b) failure of dorsiflexion of the foot is an ominous sign.
   (c) the clinical picture simulates spinal disease.
   (d) angiography is required after thrombectomy for planning reconstructive surgery.
   (e) postoperative anticoagulation until the patient is mobile is adequate.

173 Deep vein thrombosis
   (a) can be extensive without clinical signs and symptoms.
   (b) is reliably detected by radioactive I^{125} fibrinogen uptake test.
   (c) confined to the tibial veins in a patient with a history of duodenal ulcer, does not warrent anticoagulants.
   (d) involving the popliteal and more proximal veins in a patient needing surgery, requires insertion of a caval umbrella.
   (e) in the long term causes lipodermatosclerosis.

174 In fractures of long bones
   (a) involving joint surfaces usually require open reduction.
   (b) external skeletal fixation is preferable to Plaster of Paris.
   (c) due to malignant secondary deposits, internal fixation is recommended.
   (d) Volkmann's ischaemic contracture can occur in the presence of palpable distal pulses.
   (e) autogenous cortical bone graft is best used for non-union.

172 (a) **True** In atherosclerotic thrombotic occlusion because of existing collaterals, loss of function occurs later.

(b) **True** Muscles suffer ischaemia early on, hence pain precedes paraesthesia and this sign indicates significant damage. Unless the limb is revascularized promptly the damage is irreversible.

(c) **True** Nerve trauma and cerebrovascular accidents may also show similar clinical features, but these causes can be excluded if the foot pulses are absent.

(d) **False** Angiography is required preoperatively and if this is not possible it should be done during the operation in order to decide on immediate or early planned reconstruction after thrombectomy.

(e) **False** Approximately half of the postoperative deaths are caused by thrombo-embolic complications so the patient should receive from the time of operation 20–40 000 units heparin every 24 hours for 1 week followed by warfarin for 3 months.

173 (a) **True** The clinical diagnosis is also unreliable in the 30% of patients with positive clinical signs who have normal deep veins.

(b) **False** This method is sufficiently sensitive in detecting thrombosis below the inguinal ligament, but not in the femoral and pelvic veins.

(c) **True** Only 20% extend proximally into the popliteal, femoral and iliac veins and of this group, half develop pulmonary embolism. Embolism seldom occurs if thrombosis does not extend beyond the calf veins. Absolute contra-indication to drug therapy also include gastric ulcer, cerebral haemorrhage, malignant hypertension or any haemorrhagic diathesis.

(d) **True** Under local anaesthesia an umbrella-shaped filter is placed in the IVC percutaneously via the external jugular vein. The aim is to prevent large and medium sized emboli reaching the lungs.

(e) **True** These changes are thought to be the result of damage to the valves of the leg veins causing venous hypertension and exudation with fibrin accumulation around the capillaries and white cell activation.

174 (a) **True** Re-alignment of small fracture fragments near a joint is essential for restoring joint function.

(b) **False** This has the disadvantage of using pins to transfix the bone, which carries the risk of infection and is difficult to pass in other than subcutaneous bones. It is particularly useful in compound fractures where access to the wound is required.

(c) **True** Internal fixation provides early mobilization and the start of adjuvant treatment in these patients with a short life expectancy.

(d) **True** The distal pulses may be normal in the presence of significant ischaemia to muscle compartments (compartment syndrome).

(e) **False** Cancellous bone is a better material because it contains more cells with osteogenic potential. A convenient site of supply is the iliac crest.

175 In a patient with a malignant primary tumour of bone
    (a) pain at rest is the commonest presenting symptoms.
    (b) osteosarcoma is the commonest malignant tumour.
    (c) a transverse incision in a langhan line is most appropriate for the biopsy.
    (d) amputation is the curative treatment.
    (e) adjuvant chemotherapy has not improved survival.

175 (a) **True**   This can be misdiagnosed with a sprain or a sports injury but these are usually relieved by rest.

   (b) **True**   Followed by chondrosarcoma, Ewing's sarcoma and malignant fibrous histiocytoma.

   (c) **False**   The biopsy scar must be excised in block with the resection specimen. A transverse or poorly placed scar will often result in an otherwise avoidable amputation.

   (d) **False**   Limb preservation by local excision of the tumour and prosthetic reconstruction has radically changed treatment.

   (e) **False**   The 5-year survival for osteosarcoma has increased from 20 to 50% and for Ewing's sarcoma from 15 to 55%.

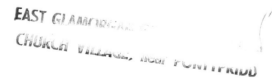

EAST GLAMORGAN

CHURCH VILLAGE, near PONTYPRIDD